Mastering Multiple Sclerosis
A Handbook of Management

Second Edition

By John K. Wolf, M.D.

Professor of Neurology
State University of New York
Health Sciences Center
Syracuse, N. Y., 13210

With:

Steven N. Fellows, M.S. (Geology), MSer
Bernice Gottschalk, B.A. (Psychology)
Bonnie Johannes, B.S. (Education), MSer
Michael Sarette, B.S. (Physical Science),
B.S. (Systems Science), MSer
Mitzi Wolf, M.S.W., C.S.W.

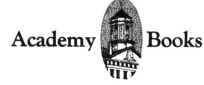

Academy Books

Copyright © 1987 by John K. Wolf

ISBN 0-914960-65-2
Library of Congress Card No. 87-70100

Printed and bound in the
United States of America
by Academy Books
Rutland, VT 05701-0757

1st Printing January 1987
2nd Printing April 1987
3rd Printing October 1987
4th Printing January 1988
5th Printing November 1988
6th Printing July 1989
7th Printing March 1990
8th Printing January 1991
9th Printing January 1992
10th Printing January 1993

Notice

The authors and publisher of this book have made every effort to ensure that all recommended treatments are in accordance with accepted medical standards at the time of publication.

Medications specified in this book may not have the specific approval of the Food and Drug Administration in regard to the indications and dosage recommended. The manufacturer's package insert is the best source of current prescribing information.

Printed instructions cannot provide individualized information that takes into account the special situation of each MSer, so your physician's recommendations may differ from those in the text. Use information from the text as an outline. Use your physician to help you discover the best treatment plan for you. In this manner you will arrive at the best possible result from the use of any medication. Do *not* use prescription medications without the assistance of your physician.

Dedication

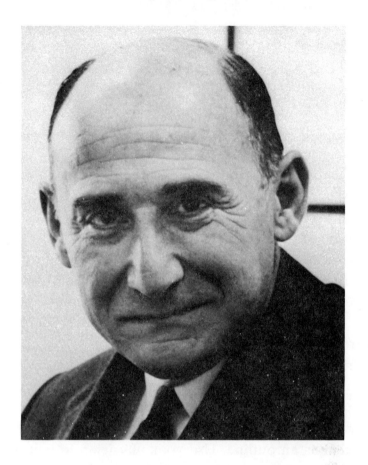

Abe B. Baker, M.D., PhD.
Regents Professor of Neurology, Emeritus
University of Minnesota

To A. B. Baker, M.D.

Dr. Baker's early efforts helped to forge the special place of neurology in American medicine. He taught precision of diagnosis and innovative management as no one else did. His passion for the Total Treatment of patients, families and disease was legend. He challenged students to aspire to excellence, always by example, occasionally even with invective!

He was already an MS doctor of great skill and compassion at a time when MSers and their families were almost universally rejected by the profession as untreatable. Dr. Baker demonstrated the value of doctoring as a prelude to the science of prescribing. Many of us, doctors and patients alike, owe him our lives.

And to Fred Krauss, Jr., MSer, 1918–1986

Fred Krauss reinforced the values of aggressive management and prolonged friendship.

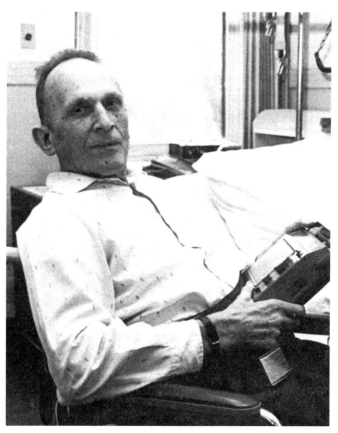

Fred Krauss, Jr., MSer.

I had just completed my residency with Dr. Baker, when I first met Fred Krauss in the Philadelphia Naval Hospital. He was a severely disabled MSer with a brilliant mind and a strong determination to overcome. Together we examined his body and his prospects. Together we began the process of rehabilitation.

After he regained lost mobility, he and I traveled to several Philadelphia area hospitals. Together, we taught medical and nursing students what we knew *then* about the diagnosis and management of multiple sclerosis. Fred became the foremost of many subsequent teacher-patients who have left their mark on my students.

Fred lived at Ingliss House in Philadelphia from 1967 through 1984, when he moved to other lodgings. While he lived at Ingliss House, he befriended fellow residents, fought for their rights and privileges and maintained close ties with his family. He saw his daughter through her PhD in clinical psychology. He reached out to families like ours and enriched our lives.

Throughout his life, Fred maintained a vivid interest in his world. He died as page proofs of this second edition arrived for correction. We shall cherish our memories of his letters and tapes, and of our times together in Philadelphia.

Table of Contents

Chapter 1

SECTION ONE

Chapter 2

Chapter 3

SECTION TWO

Chapter 4

Chapter 5

Chapter 6

Chapter 7

Chapter 8

Chapter 9

Chapter 10

Chapter 11

SECTION THREE

Chapter 12

Chapter 13

Chapter 14

Chapter 15

Chapter 16

SECTION FOUR

Chapter 17

Chapter 18

Chapter 19

Chapter 20

Acknowledgements

Bernice Gottschalk and Mike Sarette have contributed more to this volume than the reader can ever guess. They wrote chapter 15. They know the effects of disability, and have combed the text of this volume for clarity as well as errors. They were instrumental in changing the order of chapters, and in emphasizing central ideas.

Our group of MSer editors is portrayed on front and back covers of the book. I chose the editors for their experience with disability, and for their ability to examine ideas. As we wrote each chapter, the editors read them and discussed them through the mails with each author. From these discussions, many important ideas reached these pages, which could come only from such thoughtful people. Thank you, editors!

Paul Cohen, M.D., taught me how important it is for MSers to know a really fine internist. His relationship to MSers in Syracuse prompted a whole section of the chapter on doctor-patient relationships. As he read the manuscript, he accumulated the checklist of neurological concerns found on pages 295–297. This checklist could become a cornerstone of doctor-patient communications.

Marcia Ecker edited the manuscript. Her innovative use of language and syntax left me breathless, as I watched her change some of my pedestrian prose into elegant English.

Arthur Ecker, M.D., has contributed his acumen to each of my previous books. His perspective as a seasoned neurological clinician was also of great value to this text. Arthur remains a valued colleague who contributes a constant stream of interesting and useful ideas to our neurological community.

Jay Land, PhD, and his wife, Linda Land, M.S.W., both family and marriage counselors, read a number of chapters from Section Three. Their special expertise is especially to be found in Mitzi's chapters, and in Bernice and Mike's chapter on sexuality.

Many other people have examined portions of the text. MSers from many parts of the United States and from as far away as the Republic of South Africa have written to me about the previous volume, *Mastering Multiple Sclerosis*. I have gratefully recorded many of their contributions.

Bruce Dearing, PhD, Emeritus Professor of Humanities at the Upstate Medical Center, died as this manuscript neared completion. Bruce taught me to write medical information so it is understandable to English speaking people. The job was a big one. If he succeeded, readers owe him their thanks. I remember him as my professor, with fondness and admiration.

Martha Hefner and Bill Finch provided the art work for this edition, as they did for the previous one. As before, Martha devised the cover designs.

Coneco Laser Graphics set the type directly from the floppies, and devised the layout of the entire volume.

Mr. Robert Sharp and his staff at Academy Books have once more produced a book you can love to hold and read.

Many thanks to all.

Preface

Readers of the first edition of *Mastering Multiple Sclerosis,* contributed many suggestions that resulted in this completely rewritten edition. Mike Sarette and Bernice Gottschalk complained that there was no chapter on sexuality, and eventually wrote Chapter 15 themselves. Several readers asked for a chapter on pain. Chapter 8 is the result of this request. I have learned more about MS management from my own patients during the several years it has taken to produce this volume. I only wish we had made significant progress toward cure while we learned. That issue is still unresolved. Meanwhile, we can still learn management.

I have matured too. As I viewed this manuscript in its entirety, I understood clearly that the object of this book is improved mobility. I re-discovered with my patients, that despite MS, complications can be controlled. The erosion of personal independence can be postponed. Despite MS, life can remain fun.

I hope you will enjoy this volume. Above all, I hope you learn that management is worth the trouble. Keep working at it. Never give up. You are smarter than you think, and with study, you will become even smarter.

Prologue
November 15, 1982

Dear John and Mitzi,

How do you Cope? How do you deal with a diagnosis of MS? How do you struggle? These are easy questions when everything is going well. Others have had to answer them before us, and we are forced to answer them for ourselves.

The world was our oyster: beautiful, fun, joyous and filled with delight. We had four children, a lovely house in the city and summers at Cape Cod. My husband was brilliant, energetic and athletic. I would say that our marriage was made in heaven.

Then little things started to happen. My husband, who was always even tempered, began to have temper tantrums. He experienced strange sensations in his hands and legs. Our sex life, which had been joyous, changed. It was a question of who was experiencing a mental breakdown, Dick or I, so we went to see a friendly psychiatrist.

We did this for two years before Dick's symptoms and various tests indicated that he only had MS rather than a brain tumor. Which would be preferable? In many respects, it was much easier knowing the tiger you had to face rather than the unknown "something is wrong."

We both cried a lot, felt sorry for ourselves, wallowed in self pity, got angry, and then realized that these normal emotions were necessary, really vital to survival. We needed our friends for support, not pity. Dick, who had given so much of himself to others, had a hard lesson to learn. He had to become a receiver of gifts of love from others. It's nice to be a giver of kindness and a helping hand, but difficult to learn that when you receive graciously you allow others to be givers, and in turn are still giving.

I had to learn to change roles. The head of the household, mechanic, electrician, mother, bookkeeper, plumber, chauffeur, breadwinner, all were mine now. I had been a "kept woman" because Dick had always done everything so capably. His was a hard act to follow. I went back to school and became a teacher for selfish reasons. I liked to vacation all summer on the beach, and teaching allowed me to do it.

I also learned to do all sorts of things, such as giving shots—"You can do this, Verah, you're strong," said the physician. My reply was "You've got to be kidding! I'm not strong, whatever that means!" I remember saying to Dick once, that I was never cut out to be a nurse. This is not my calling! His reply: "Well, I was never cut out to be a patient!" That shut me up. We have worked together at our unchosen avocations.

It was difficult, too, to learn that you could get angry at your spouse who was in a wheelchair. Just because he couldn't walk didn't mean he had an invisible shield around him that allowed him to be cantankerous and nasty. We all have bad days.

One of the things we and our kids have learned is that if this is the worst day of your life, then tomorrow has to be better, because you have just lived through the worst one.

When Dick first learned that he had MS, he wrote a letter to all his colleagues at the university. He said he wanted their continued friendship, not their pity. He also wrote a letter to each of his children, who were 10, 8, 6 and 4 at the time, stating that his dreams for their future would have to be modified because of MS. He said that they would have to grow up faster and accept more responsibilities. They accepted his challenge. It hasn't been easy, but it's a fact that the finest steel is tempered in the hottest fire.

How do you cope? You take one day at a time. You pray. You cry buckets if you have to, and then you get up, blow your nose and say that tomorrow has to be better. You joy that you are still together. You lean on your true friends for support when necessary. You know that somewhere, sometime, there will be a cause and a cure for MS and others will not have to face this ordeal.

How do you struggle? You hang on and let go. You love and joy in the thought that this is the best of all possible worlds. It's not trite to say that you glory in all the sunsets and sunrises. The following poem has helped me in my struggle:

Invitation to Serenity
by Vivian T. Pomeroy

When we are tired with the work we have to do, or feel
    unequal to it,
When we dully wonder about its being worthwhile,
When our pleasures, so easily taken, communicate no
    happiness to the heart,
When we are forgetting about our own faults or the faults of
    other people,
When one day repeats another and we pine for some change, we
    know not what,
Then, may the voices of our own heart's courage, and of age
    long wisdom, call us to their hospitality.

When there is sound and fury all around signifying little or
  nothing,
When the past derides us with remembered failures, and we
  think we are never to be rid of them,
When the future seems more a menace than a hope,
When we feel that at our worst it will not matter much, and
  at our best it will not really count,
When we are a prey to fears because we cannot guard against
  a chance, and a slight thing happening would lay us low,
Then may we receive, each for himself, the comforting
  assurance: *In quietness and confidence shall be your strength!*

Hope this helps,

Verah

Verah

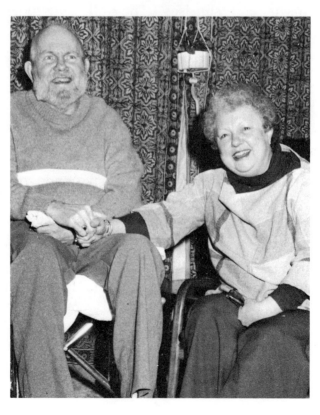

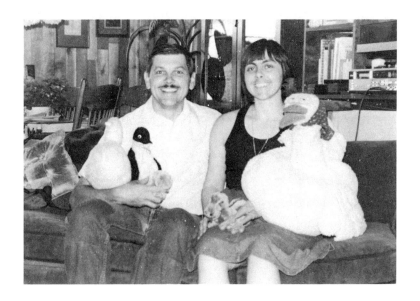

August 16, 1985

Dear John,

Suddenly, as my thoughts and reactions to the *Second Edition* gel, I'm obsessed with management. I'm like a kid with a new toy. The box it came in fascinates me for hours! As I learn management techniques, this disease is whittled from overwhelming and terrifying to a size I can handle. You offer us MSers a choice, or choices in managing our disease. It's like finding a road map with all kinds of roads and towns and all, and I'm in one town and need to get to another. There's a main road—say the interstate—but there are also alternative routes that will do the job. They do it differently, but I still can *get* there.

I'm glad you left in the part about dragging sand into the house with the wheelchair. That's a special enticement for me to keep on living! We have finally gotten rain—days of it. I nearly drug in a worm with the wheelchair yesterday!

As always,

Bonnie

Bonnie Johannes

Chapter One

An Introduction to Multiple Sclerosis
By John K. Wolf

From the black hole of Hell
To the open sun on the mountain,
This, my journey of the past four years.

I feel I am recovering from a terrible accident.
The implosion of diagnosis: Shock.
My body functions on automatic.
While deep inside I try to stop the bleeding.
Disbelief. I cry. I scream.

Someone I love is dead. She's never coming back.
Do I want to live or not?
Yes. No! No? Well, Maybe. I'll try once more.
God, it's gonna be a lot of work, starting from scratch.

Life stays. It's just a glimmer in the dark,
But I grab on.
One thing leads to another, and then another,
Then there's more light than dark, more healed than
broken.

I'm well enough to go home now.
I'll take what's left of me,
And begin again on the new me.

Bonnie Johannes
September, 1985

1

Are you newly come to MS, still fearful? This book is for you, to banish despair through knowledge. You will no longer be unschooled when you have read these pages. Or are you an old timer, already skilled in the wiles of management? We write also for you. This second edition of *Mastering Multiple Sclerosis* contains ideas from MSers across this country and from as far away as Africa, who have written in response to the first. We have used their ideas, and we have learned a few things ourselves. Even old timers can learn a trick or two, to solve a problem we may already understand.

So read to learn that MS is not an enormous burden set upon your shoulders, but a series of smaller problems with solutions that partially, or sometimes wholly circumvent. Make a firm decision to live each day for itself, and to cope daily with anything that comes along. If you decide, as we have, that mobility is your chief priority, pursue mobility. You can establish other priorities: a happy productive family life, relief from pain, and relief from embarrassment when body functions work off schedule. You can *decide* how to pursue your profession as well as your roles of parent, son, daughter, nephew, aunt or friend. You can *decide in advance* to use all your ability to learn new tricks to keep yourself and your loved ones happy.

The lifestyles of MSers parallel the lifestyles of physically healthy people in success and failure, in joy and sadness. Your fellow MSers are living their lives as parents, spouses, business people, housewives, engineers. Some of them live in nursing homes; others completely alone, but they manage, as other solitary people do. Today you may think you are at the end of the road. Chances are that you are not, and that you will discover successful ways to cope.

This is a handbook, designed to stay on your bedside table, or perhaps to live in the bathroom, handy for daily reference. Take notes in the margins. Modify our ideas to fit your needs. Then remember: This is just the second edition. It is improved because others wrote to us. Help us make a third edition more informative, more fun to read.

WHAT IS MS?

We know the cause of MS *symptoms*: MS plaques in the central nervous system. But no one really knows what causes MS *plaques*. Plaques are local areas of damage in the brain and spinal cord. You will read about plaques and you can see a picture of them in Figs. 18-1 and 18-2, page 329. We do not know how plaques form, nor what determines their placement. We do not know why some people develop many plaques in a short time, and have rapidly progressive disability, while others remain essentially stable over many years. We know that many MSers have abnormal laboratory tests, but we have no idea which are related to the cause, and which merely to the presence of MS.

We do know that MS is not contagious. Your mother-in-law will not catch it from you, nor your spouse, nor your friends. If someone you know is still worried about *that* question, lay the worry to rest.

What is the Cure for MS?

Without known cause, there is no cure. Throughout their lives, MSers are bombarded with information. Everyone wants to help: friends, neighbors, newspapers, legitimate practitioners familiar with the scientific literature, and people you don't even know, who may approach you on the street! We all continue to hope that this year's answer may finally be the right one. Quack practitioners wait at every turn to raise false hopes and fleece the gullible. When information comes your way, you will be tempted to spend your money and your hope. I encourage you to do it, if you must, but read Chapter 20 first. It might help you to identify and avoid the quacks. Someday we shall find the right answer. When we do, we shall all breathe a sigh of relief and get to the business of cure. Until then, beware of false prophets.

So Why Should You Bother with this Book?

Because ideas presented in subsequent chapters can improve your life. The first section introduces you to MS, to the book, and to *Mobility*, the central issue of management. Section Two deals with management of MS symptoms. Section Three suggests ways to manage your relationships with the people in your life. In 1992, management is your chief weapon. When new symptoms develop, they can usually be managed. Each chapter by each author teaches you moment-to-moment details about management practices that have worked for other MSers. We have used the techniques we describe, and we have exposed our ideas to MSer experts in symptom management before our words reached the printed page. Techniques in this volume can neither remove plaques from your brain nor change the course of MS in your nervous system. But they can help you achieve some ambitions that might otherwise have miscarried through ignorance.

There is *always* management. Your legs won't walk? Have you found the best available wheelchair so you can get around anyway? If not, now is the time to get crackin'! If you have, go ahead. Be mobile despite bad legs. Go out and attack the problems of your world, as others attack the problems of theirs.

MSers who understand their disease, like professionals who understand their jobs, are more effective, and have more fun in life. When the MS or the profession changes, capable people are ready for new ideas. Indeed, successful MSers come to regard themselves as professionals in the business of *management*.

This book *preaches* management. We authors have learned that if a new symptom is attacked immediately, complications are reduced and life is improved. We want you to learn that lesson.

MS is no fun. No one envies you your disease. But no illness is fun, and many people, young and old, have lingering illnesses, some much worse than MS. By contrast, successful management *can* be fun. Readers who once were confined and then found a way to rejoin life, remember such triumphs with pleasure.

Section Four of this volume discusses medical ideas: Anatomy, Diagnosis, Prognosis, Quackery and Research. In these chapters, I hope you will find answers to questions like:

"Why do I have double vision and loss of feeling?"
"How do you know I have MS?"
"Did I find the right doctor to take care of me?"
"Do I need a second opinion, or a third?"
"How much disability can I expect to have in five years?"

Originally, I put Section Four at the front of the book. The issues of anatomy, accuracy of diagnosis and prognosis are of first importance to my professional life. I thought they were of prime importance to MSers as well. But my editors convinced me that for MSers, *management* is the first issue. So Section Four comes last. Thoughtful, successful MSers *insisted* that a book for MSers be written that way.

We end with a glossary of words used in this volume, and an index that is as complete as we could make it. If you study this book, you will find your time has been well spent.

ACCOMPLISHMENT

Reading this, one might think that management consists of a series of battles won against the various symptoms of MS. It does. But management is also a series of battles lost. Normal aging is also a series of battles lost. But those who age well lose their battles one at a time, and then go on to other activities. MSers must also plan such losing battles. But with MS, the losses occur at a younger age. The pain of youthful disability is that MSers' minds are young, but their bodies have aged. MSers and their friends have the mental vitality of youth, but while the friends have physical vitality as well, the MSer's capacity is limited. This hurts, and there is no local anesthetic to stop the pain.

One of our editors taught school for years from her wheelchair. Eventually, she found that she no longer had energy for week after week of teaching. So she retired. She has kept her mind active, but her body refuses her command. Even so, she continues to use her physical capacities as well as possible. In a recent letter, she expressed her pain better than I ever could.

"Dear Dr. Wolf,

"I'm sure you are getting many phone calls and much mail due to our early summer weather this year. I'm feeling fine physically, but my state of mind is not very good.

"I am experiencing new emotions (for me) and I don't like it. All my friends are moving on—career advancement—and I'm stopped. Jealous, that's me. They talk about work. I listen, but I can't contribute. I feel that life is at a standstill. I'm only 34 and want more, but . . . .

"To overcome, I'm calling elderly individuals but it's just not the same.

"I'll see you in a couple of weeks. Maybe my spirits will be brighter then."

There is no comfort for those feelings as long as the mind is 34 and the body is 68. Acceptance comes to some healthy people as they age, and to some MSers as their disease progresses. Search for acceptance. It can give you a measure of peace. But while you search, continue to volunteer and to work, to call older individuals and to visit your fellow MSers when they are sick. There is more to life than acceptance.

Take from this book ideas about management, about success against heavy odds and about living. Your success will depend more on your personality and spirit, than upon this new disease and its symptoms. If you are determined and inventive, nothing can keep you down. If you have been only modestly inventive, learn from your colleagues. Absorb other people's successes into your own life. If you are a senior MSer with years of experience, or a junior MSer who is exceptionally able to cope, spread your success among the less successful. Let us all work to benefit the entire MS community, the

wider community of disabled people, and the still wider
community of humankind. Make this world better for
your passage. We leave nothing behind but the results
of our work.

"MSer"

We do not need MS plaques in the brain to suffer MS
with a spouse, parent, friend, or patient. Although
"MSer" refers primarily to anyone who has MS, all of us
who are affected by MS are, to varying degrees, MSers.

Some readers have had trouble with the term
"MSer," and struggle to find a better one. "Persons who
have MS" repeated ten thousand times in a few hundred pages would be incredibly clumsy. "MS Victims"
is worse. "MS patients" makes no sense. MSers are
patients for only a few minutes every few months for a
periodic visit to a physician, or for a few weeks if they
are hospitalized. The rest of the time they are people,
living their lives in many different and sometimes
exciting ways.

Some people have trouble with "MSer" because they
want to avoid a label. "MSer" is a noun, not a label. It
describes the only thing that all "Persons Who Have
MS" really *do* have in common.

Last, the term "MSer" travels in good company. If
you meet someone between the ages of 13 and 19, does
the word "teenager" come to mind? What do you call a
person who belongs to 4-H, or who runs sweating and
panting past your home, dressed in fancy shoes and
shorts, wearing a sweatband around the forehead? They
are 4-H-ers and jogg-ers. But each person has myriad
other characteristics and abilities which can be described appropriately when they are used.

Use the term "MSer" with comfort, but also refer to all the other characteristics of MSers as they become important. Many nouns and adjectives accurately describe the Persons who have been Editors and the MSers who are Authors of this volume. They are also graduate students, a computer systems analyst, teachers, housewives, middle aged, retired, volunteers, disabled and many more. For the purpose of this volume they are Editors and Authors. I chose them because, as MSers, they are experts in what they do.

You call it Courage,
And are amazed that I am out and about.

I say Why not?
It may be more complicated for me,
But you are here. Why shouldn't I be, too?

Bonnie Johannes
October, 1985

SECTION ONE

Mobility and Access:

the Chief Goals
of Management

Introduction

Management means mobility. Everything we do, healthy or sick, either promotes our access to the world, or detracts from it. If we cannot go out, if we are confined in any way, we are by that degree deprived of the fun of life, and the excitement of doing what we wish.

All of us must promote the idea that disabled people are no different from anyone else, except that some body functions misfire. Some people travel in wheelchairs. Some live in wheelchairs. But they are not confined to wheelchairs any more than physically healthy people are confined to their automobiles, as long as they have mobility as a result.

The next two chapters present ideas to get you started. In this chapter we examine specific aids to walking and riding. In the next chapter, Steve Fellows considers modifications to your community, your house and your transportation. As you consider our ideas, examine your own living arrangements, your financial resources, your family and yourself. Think of innovative ways to improve mobility in your own surroundings, with an eye to your future physical condition.

Approach your disability piecemeal: a weak ankle, a tight spastic right leg, bladder symptoms that require attention. To one degree or another, each can be improved or circumvented. As you attack each symptom, you will improve your total condition. If instead, you view MS as a single enormous burden, you may be tempted to give up, because it is too much to take on all at once. But you are into this for the long haul. Decide now that you will become an expert in management, so that you may improve your mobility for the rest of your life.

Chapter 2
Aids to Mobility
By John K. Wolf

Effective management allows MSers to move about at home and travel away from home, despite physical disability. The goal is easily met in early stages of MS, but becomes more difficult as disability progresses. Maintenance of mobility often requires help from other people. Even severely disabled MSers can remain mobile despite progressive physical symptoms. Some even travel widely.

AIDS TO AMBULATION

After reading this chapter, editor Richard Carrington commented that MS is a progressive illness. It is important to acquire aids to mobility early, so they will remain useful for a long time. I have two favorite aids to walking: the forearm (Canadian) crutch and the ankle splint. As Dick Carrington points out, they will be more useful if you get them when you first need them. If a brace or Canadian crutches become inadequate, a wheelchair is indispensable for active living.

Grandfather's Cane

In our hospital, the obstetricians have their offices near the waiting room, surgeons next and neurologists at the far end of the hall. People have to walk farther to me than to anyone else. Usually when people begin to stumble or stagger, they hunt up an old cane that's been left in the attic since Grandfather's time. If there is no cane, or if the attic is too crowded to find *anything*, a spouse or friend become handy supports. I recognize disability caused by gait disturbance as they come down the hall to my office. This is my signal to prescribe a Canadian crutch, because under most circumstances Grandfather's cane is inadequate.

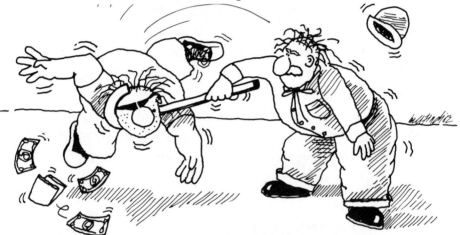

Fig. 2-1. Unsurpassed for felling muggers.

Grandfather acquired his cane toward the end of an active life, because his arthritis made it hard for him to climb the hill to the barn. Grandfather had a powerful grip and an excellent cerebellum. MSers often have weakness of grip and imbalance. With his powerful grip, Grandfather could flick his cane where he needed it for support. On his infrequent trips to New York City, Grandfather found his cane unsurpassed for felling muggers in Central Park (Fig. 2-1).

The cane was fine for Grandfather, but MSers often find it of little help. If grip is weak the cane provides no support in a fall. It gets in the way and may actually cause trouble rather than prevent it. Grandfather's cane is useful only for MSers who have a powerful grip and merely need support for weak legs.

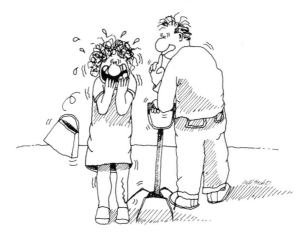

Fig. 2-2. Taking the shinbone of a passing pedestrian.

Four-Point Cane

Four-point canes reduce the wobble of Grandfather's cane, but the mechanics of this cane are only slightly better than Grandfather's. The weakened hand is still at the wrong end of the long fulcrum. The four little feet do not hold the ground much better than the regular cane. A weak hand and arm at the top cannot move the heavy tip quickly and accurately enough to prevent disaster.

Consider also the effect of a four-point cane on a person who has just purchased one in order to remain mobile. As he strides confidently along, the little feet stick out about a foot from his side, taking with them the shinbone of a passing pedestrian (Fig. 2-2), with predictable results. (Fig. 2-3)

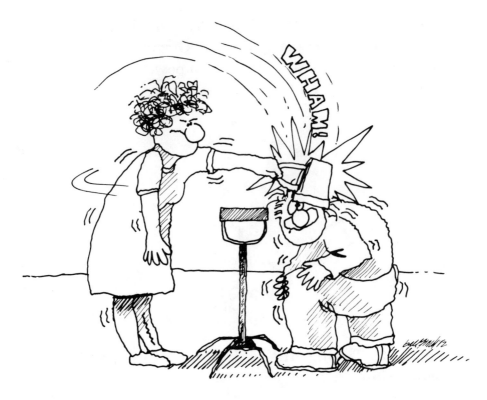

Fig. 2-3. Not a pleasant beginning to newly-won mobility.

Avoid the four-point cane!

Forearm Crutch

MSers with imbalance, spasticity and loss of power in arms and legs need support up high where the imbalance is. On the ground the appliance should be lithe, easy to place and fast to move. The Canadian crutch fits that description precisely. It is a sturdy cane with an extension that clasps the forearm firmly. The handgrip provides good support even if the hand's grip is weak.

If you begin to fall while using a Canadian crutch you can move the tip rapidly for support and lean on it. You can even get a Canadian crutch with an ice tong so you may go for a promenade in Central New York snowstorms (Fig. 2-4).

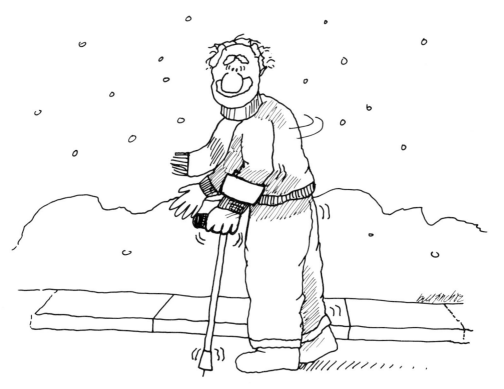

Fig. 2-4. The ice tong for winter promenades.

Editor, Barbara Shetron has found a perfect compromise for the MSer who wants a forearm crutch above and four-footed support down below. She has a Canadian crutch with four little feet on the bottom and a rubber junction that allows the feet to lie flat on uneven surfaces (Fig. 2-5). She swears she has never been *"wham!ed"* under the severest provocation.

Bonnie Johannes replaced the plastic handgrips on her Canadian crutches with "Grab-Ons®," rough surfaced, dense foam hand grips sold for motor cycles. She

says they are vastly more comfortable than the origi-
nals.

When should you buy the crutch? Probably right
now. If you need to hold onto furniture and walls *inside*,
then buy the crutch to use when you go *out*. Buy it when
you first need it, not after you have to hang onto
someone else to get around or after you have fallen and
hurt yourself. Consider whether you wouldn't do better
with a pair rather than a single crutch.

Go to a Physician's and Hospital Supply store and ask
to try their forearm crutches. Look at the various styles
and see which you like. Spend time walking around the
store with them. Perhaps they will lend you a pair to use
for several days before you actually buy them. Talk to
MSers who already have them. Talk to your physical
therapist and your doctor to get their ideas. Then ask for
a specific prescription to fill your need.

Editor's Note:

"Put in something about how to find the
proper length of cane or crutch. We recently
tried to buy a pair of 'Shetron Specials' and the
salesman kept saying the pair in stock were
long enough, when they obviously were not.

We're sure this happens all the time."

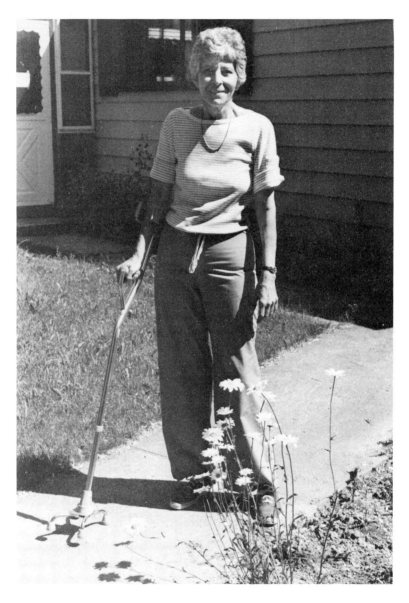

Fig. 2-5. The "Shetron Special" provides four-point support below, and assured balance above.

As Mike and Bernice discovered, salesmen are there to sell, not to take care of *you*. Another of my MSers was sold a set of ready-made ankle splints, despite a poor fit in the store. The salesman assured her the splints were adjustable. But her legs were fat, and the splint did not adjust enough to fit.

When you begin research into a wheelchair, the salesman who doesn't sell the new style wheelchairs may indicate that they are only for basketball games. Rubbish! If a basketball player can get around a fast court more quickly and more safely, why should you settle for less at home or at work?

Remember. It's your money and your mobility. Don't buy anything unless you know it's right.

Ankle Splint

The cock-up ankle splint is the second highly effective tool for the walking MSer with ankle weakness. MSers lose power in the three major muscles that control the ankle: the anterior tibial muscle to lift the toes, and the peroneus and posterior tibial muscles to stabilize the ankle on the sides.

Anterior tibial muscle weakness results in a foot drop that allows the toes to catch on rugs, door jambs and steps. If the toes are not supported to clear these obstructions you may stumble and fall headlong.

The peroneus muscles support the outside of the ankle. Peroneus weakness allows the ankle to collapse outward, and cause a fall or sprain if you step on uneven ground or tread on a toy truck in the night.

The posterior tibial muscle supports the inside of the ankle. Perhaps because the other foot is there for support, it generally is of less importance than the peroneus muscles, but if the posterior tibial is weak the ankle still may drop you to the ground.

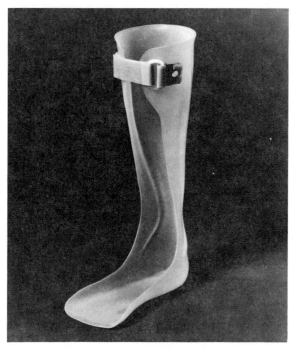

Fig. 2-6. Plastic ankle brace. The generic splint for people with generic legs. Photograph courtesy of the Ohio Truss Corporation.

MSers usually know that the ankle is weak because they have felt it turn under them as they walk. Some have already fallen and broken something before the doctor knows anything is wrong. If you think an ankle is weak, ask your neurologist or your physical therapist to test it for you and show you and family members how to test it at home.

At the first sign of weakness, learn muscle strengthening exercises. Do them frequently each day to delay progression of the weakness. Exercise will be good for your muscles and focus your attention on ankle function, so you will be alert when the ankle begins to collapse.

If the exercises do not keep the ankle strong, buy the brace. It fits right inside the shoe and cocks the toes up automatically to prevent stumbles. It supports the ankle on the sides to prevent sprains. It weighs only a few ounces and the benefit to gait is impressive.

Splints molded specially to the shape of your own leg and foot cost several hundred dollars, but mass-produced splints are available for about $70.00. I am uncertain which to recommend. If you are very fat or very thin, if you are exceptionally tall or short, or if your ankles alternately swell and shrink, order a splint that is specially molded to your leg. However if you have "generic legs," the mass-produced generic splints will work very well. They come in three different sizes. To a limited degree they can be molded to fit better.

Perhaps you may consider an even simpler device. Roy Bloom, from Union Gap, Washington, sent us an illustration of an ankle splint suspended from a Velcro® band around the leg, just below the knee. Attached to it, by monofilament line, is an elastic band of sufficient power to lift the toe. From the elastic, a second monofilament line is attached to the toe of the shoe. Roy reports he uses moccasins, as the only footwear that allows comfortable shuffling without tripping, and the monofilament passes easily through a snap swivel installed on the toe. Incidentally, Roy recommends Velcro® for many other attaching jobs at home, like buttons on sleeves, collars and pants.

The price for this splint is right. Roy suggests a dollar per shoe. However, it must be attached and re-attached with awkward fingers unless you have installed a snap swivel on every shoe in the house. Since the life of an elastic band is limited, plan to re-make your home-made splint frequently.

Roy Bloom's splint does not protect against ankle weakness on the sides. If, in addition to simple foot drop, your ankle has a tendency to collapse inward or outward, consider your safety first. Spend the money for a plastic brace.

Like Canadian crutches, ankle splints are most useful when ankle weakness first endangers gait. Ankle splints retain limited value to the wheeler with weak ankles, who needs to keep the toes cocked up to transfer. Get your ankle muscles tested. If they are slightly weak, get them strengthened with active P.T. If they are dangerously weak, get them supported.

Sure Grip Plastic Dot Gloves May Help Your Hands

Improve mobility of your hands, while you're at it. Bonnie Johannes, sent us a pair of Sure Grip gloves from Jeffers Handbell Supply, inc., Carillon Park, R.D. 2 Box 159, Irmo, SC, 29063-9063, catalog No.: 30PDNS. They are made of light cotton fabric with little plastic nubbins on the palm side. Their close fit improves a weak, incoordinated grip. They are designed for light work, like turning pages while reading, not pushing wheelchair rims or pulling weeds. The cost: $3.50 per pair, plus $1.00 shipping and handling charge *per order*. Specify small, medium, large or extra large size.

WHEELCHAIR

During the past few years a bewildering array of new manual and electric wheelchairs has arrived on the market. Previously life was simpler. There were only two manufacturers and the products were so similar that one could choose on the basis of price alone. Now you must consider extreme variations in function, weight, engineering, color and appearance.

For over thirty years the standard has been Everest and Jennings®*. At one time they manufactured the only line of really good wheelchairs and backed up their product with nationwide service and excellent repair policies. They are still a standard for the industry. You should investigate E. & J.® when you look at chairs.

Rolls Invacare® invaded the E. & J. market by producing a chair that was just as light and just as sturdy. Many people have turned to Rolls for their chairs. Investigate Rolls.

In the spring of 1984, a new concept in wheelchairs reached Syracuse from California and revolutionized my notion of a functional chair for MSers. These new chairs have many features of racing bikes, which is no accident in the case of the Quadra®. The founders of that company were a bike manufacturer and a paraplegic wheeler. Dissatisfied with available technology, they designed their own product.

These new style chairs have little resemblance to the boxy chairs of the past. They "move out" while they still stand in the sales window. The frame of welded aircraft metal comes in numerous colors. Wheels have quick-release hubs like racing bikes. This allows the chair to be instantly dismantled for a car trip. These new chairs are so light, you may even decide to toss yours in the car without taking it apart.

The balance and movement are also different from

---

* Note: Addresses for wheelchair manufacturers may be found on page 34.

24

the old style chairs. Nearly all the rider's weight rests on the bicycle tires in the rear. The small front tires carry almost none. These light front wheels make little impression as they roll across the pile of a rug or through the tomato patch.

The chairs move rapidly with minimum effort. The rear wheels can be cambered in at the top to provide better leverage for the hands and arms coming down along them to the push rim. While the camber adds several inches to the over-all width of the chair, this feature also adds zip to the chair's movement.

By moving the rear axles to different positions, the wheeler can raise or lower the body of the chair and move the wheel forward or backward along the center of gravity to fit specific needs of body weight and balance. These chairs come with an anti-tip device that many active wheelers eventually discard. You should definitely use this safety feature *at least* while you learn to manage the chair. Get the large semipneumatic front wheels too, for improved mobility outside the house. Tiny front wheels look sporty, but they work best only on the basketball court.

If you do not investigate these new chairs before you buy, you will have missed an opportunity. By the time you read this section, several other manufacturers may produce just what you want, so do your research and buy the best chair you can find.

Then buy your wheelchair early. Don't wait till you require it simply to cross your living room. If you can still walk a mile without trouble, walk. But when you need to walk three miles, or when you want to go to the

State Fair for a whole day, use the wheelchair to get you there. Then enjoy the trip.

Buying Your Chair

If you have decided to buy your chair early so you can use it to remain active, it must work well for many years and adapt to your changing needs. Accept a chair from the lady down the block if it's inexpensive, but plan to keep it only as a spare. Use it consistently only while you research the field. Don't spend good money on bad transportation. Get a top of the line chair.

If you plan to use it inside and outside the house, you must have balloon tires. This creates a problem. MSers with severe weakness of arms may require hard rubber tires, to roll more easily across rugs indoors. In that case, if you can afford it, buy an electric for outside, a manual for inside.

Balloon tires bring in more sand when you come in from the outside. But since you bought the chair to remain active, that sand is no longer dirt. It remains on the floor as one more evidence of *grit* in your response to disability. You could not possibly have brought sand into the living room, had you not been truly living.

Three further options may be important, if they are not included as standard equipment on your chair. Removable arm rests allow easy transfers from the side of the chair. This would be much more difficult if the arms could not be removed. Most chairs offer a variety of arm rest styles. If you want a different style next year, you can switch. Or you can remove the arms completely for improved mobility.

Heel loops protect your feet from falling off the back of the foot rests, even if there is no weakness. They add significantly to comfort.

Brake handle extensions are available for some chairs, which make for easier manipulation of the brake levers.

Manual wheelchairs are expensive. Electrics cost even more. Do not simply go out and buy a chair or ask your doctor to prescribe one. Do your homework. Make the rounds of Physician and Hospital Supply stores and look at their chairs. Get catalogs and price lists for comparison. Look at advertisements in magazines like *Accent on Living* (1)* and *Paraplegia News* (3).* Send for manufacturer's literature. Be aware that brand new companies may fail in a few years, while well established corporations are more likely to be around to provide needed repairs and service. However, it may be worth the risk if a new product is exactly what you need at the right price, so look carefully.

Once you have learned about styles and prices of wheelchairs, collect ideas from MSers with experience living in their own chairs. Talk with your physical therapist and doctor who have experience prescribing them. Take home several chairs on trial so you can get a feel for their action. If your supplier is uninterested in lending you a chair, go somewhere else to buy. You won't plunk down $1500 or more without knowing precisely what you will get for your money.

Before you write up the final order, *be certain you have been properly measured* to get the right sized chassis, proper width and depth of seat, and proper height of back rest. Consider all the options available and decide which are important to you. Then be certain your physician has written a prescription that precisely de-

---

* Note: Addresses for these periodicals may be found on page 35.

scribes the brand name, style, size and all accessories you have ordered.

Consider the Electrics

Sometime, you will probably want an electric to maintain mobility. Does your job require traveling around in the building? Ride in comfort. Do you like to tour the shopping malls? Take your electric. Buy it with the same care you used shopping for the manual. You want to be happy with it when it comes.

Mike Sarette and Bernice Gottschalk, who also wrote Chapter 15, have published an article on three-wheeled electric vehicles (2). You may find it in your public library or in the library of a local independent living center. The three-wheeled carts are a different breed from the standard electric wheelchairs. They move differently, and feel different. You should definitely try out both the standard electrics and the three-wheeled carts as you research the question of powered mobility.

Are you avoiding the purchase of an electric wheelchair or cart because you are concerned that pampering yourself will make you go soft? That is an unwarranted fear. Physically healthy people still use their legs even though they travel around in automobiles. MSers can continue to use their muscles even though they travel around in electric wheelchairs. The electric will allow you to *decide* how to use your energies each day, and will take you to places you could not visit unassisted. On bad days, MSers who usually use the manual can continue to be mobile with the electric. Once you have the electric, continue with your active physical therapy program to keep yourself fit while you keep moving.

Like other aids to mobility the electric has its best use for certain degrees of disability and certain activities. It should be available when it is first needed to keep you active, interest*ed* and interest*ing*. Beg, borrow, buy or steal your electric early, when it first gets hard to keep active in the manual. If you do not, you will get it too late—after abandoning cherished activities. People do not go back to doing things they have abandoned, even when the situation changes to make it easier again. Get the electric for transportation. Get it early and use it. Arrive rested on the electric, so that you can use your physical capabilities to the utmost and still be comfortable, while you actively enjoy your life.

"We have Often Thought that with Unlimited Funds, being disabled wouldn't be all that bad," wrote Bernice Gottschalk and Mike Sarette after they read this section.

> "Most people in America don't have to choose between medical care for their children and food for the rest of the family, thank God. But people in America often have to make painful choices about how to allocate family resources. Is it really always better to get the best wheelchair the first time if it is needed for only occasional use? That may mean giving up other things that can be equally important. People are going to do what they have to do regardless of what you say in this book. We think they will be more likely to get the wheelchair early if you concede that a piece of used and less than ideal equipment may nevertheless be a real boon and provide lots of joyful mobility."

I don't know the answer to this challenge, either.

29

Chronic illness *is* a financial burden, and no family has enough money to do all the things that must be done. My plea to you is to search through your priorities and to keep mobility at the top of your list. Forego some things in order to remain active. Don't stay home. If a second-hand piece of equipment will do the trick, use it. Just don't plan to keep it forever, and do reject everything that reduces your mobility.

DEPRESSION DESTROYS MOBILITY

Mine is a varied neurological practice. I see people who have become disabled from accidents, from seizure disorder, from the complications of many diseases. Many of these people are young, but almost without exception when I recognize and treat depression, I am talking with an MSer. Depression among MSers is more than a response to disability. It represents the placement of MS plaques somewhere in the depths of the brain.

This is important because, although depression is eminently treatable, MSers, families and physicians often fail to recognize it. If depression is damaging your life, read no further till you have studied Chapter 7. If the description of depressed life resembles your own — *please!*— get treatment now with generic Elavil® or, if Elavil is not indicated for some reason, with another effective antidepressant medication, and begin to live again.

Then come back to this chapter and see what you can make of tomorrow.

PHYSICAL THERAPY

Physical therapy is important for maintaining power and mobility. Specific exercises improve specific muscle function. Gait training improves walking. Physical therapists can suggest alternative ways of doing things when the going gets rough. Physical therapists can measure you and specify sizes of wheelchair and walking crutch to fit your body.

Physical therapists are professionals. They spend years mastering their art, so one small section of a single chapter cannot teach you about P.T. Ask for a physical therapy consultation to learn now how to improve your stamina and mobility. Your time and money will be well spent if you find a competent person to teach you.

Remember that physical therapy is not something the therapist does *to* you. Physical therapy techniques must be learned so they can go home with you for daily use. Once you begin physical therapy, it becomes a way of life. If you have enough stamina, plan to spend at least 15 minutes one or more times a day on your exercises.

Many other exercises can be done at intervals during the day. Are you working at your desk or sitting in front of the TV? That is a perfect place to do ankle, knee and some hip exercises. Are you putting the dishes away after supper? Arm strengthening exercises make the chore more interesting and improve shoulder strength at the same time. Are you walking down the corridor at work, or from livingroom to bathroom at home? That is a perfect place to practice precise stepping and balance exercises. Indeed, you can set up an increasingly difficult gait-training course in the kitchen or hallway at home to train your legs and body in the most effective use of balance. Then use it every time you walk down the hall. Do as much P.T. during the day as you can without aggravating exhaustion. Do it consistently. Do it continuously. You should be tired at the end of the day but not worn out for the next three.

It is extra hard to do P.T. on bad days and during periods of exacerbation. During these times, strive for maintenance. Active P.T. will not damage your nervous system even during an attack, but it will help to keep you in shape so you can take best advantage of the coming remission or of the better day tomorrow.

Do not expect instant results. It usually takes several months of regular exercise for muscles to develop more power and stamina, whether you are MSer or physically healthy. Balance and walking may improve rapidly if you are doing gait training exercises that do not depend on raw power. Gait and balance will continue to improve afterward as power improves. Once you reach a plateau, continue to work to keep yourself at the best possible level of function.

One caution: Use judgment about gait training exercises. If you practice complex stepping and balance exercises on downtown streets, you may be home late for supper, after explaining yourself to little men in white coats!

"You still don't have a section on swimming?"
—asked Don Finster. "You should tell your readers, so they can get the benefit of the exercise!" So I asked Don to write a short segment for you, as encouragement to join a regular swimming group near you.

"I re-discovered swimming in 1983. While I was on a vacation in Puerto Rico, I spent an average of 5 hours a day in the hotel swimming pool. When I came home, I went to the local YMCA and began to work regularly with a physical therapist.

"The water makes my body buoyant. I can do exercises in the pool I never could do on land, such as deep knee bends against the pool side, push-ups on the drain gutter, and leg extensions.

"Regular swimming for the past 18 months has been better medicine for me than any doctor could have prescribed. I swim for two hours, six days a week. Usually I swim about a mile per day. This is the equivalent of jogging four miles, which I never could do in my condition. I swim most of the distance under water, coming up only for breath, but I am developing a floating backstroke as well.

"Swimming relaxes tense muscles and nerves. I have built up my endurance. My swimming and breathing techniques have improved. My physical condition is better. I have never felt so well!

How could I give you a better recommendation than that? Don's experience is duplicated by many MSers. If you plan regular exercise, swimming is one of the best ways to get it. Have fun while you keep fit!

WANT INTERNATIONAL MOBILITY? WRITE MIUSA!

Mobility International U.S.A. has a newsletter and fascinating publications for mobility-minded people. Their book, *A World of Options* ($11.00 for MIUSA members, $13.00 non-members) has information about international exchange programs, international work camps, travel ideas for U.S. and foreign travel and a series of personal essays from members. They report studies in Europe and South— and Central America, Work Camp and Peace Corps experiences, and even hitch hiking through New Zealand by wheelchair! For more information, write: Mobility International U.S.A., P.O. Box 3551, Eugene, Oregon, 97403. Or call: (503) 343-1284.

Wheelchair Manufacturers:

Everest and Jennings®
3233 East Mission Oaks Blvd.
Camarillo, Ca. 93010
(805) 987-6911

Invacare Corporation®
1200 Taylor St., P.O. Box 4028
Elyria, Oh. 44036
(216) 329-6000

Motion Designs, inc. (The Quicky®)
2842 Business Park Ave.
Fresno, Ca. 93727
(209) 292-2171

Quadra® Wheelchairs, Inc.
31117 Via Colinas
Westlake Village, Ca. 91362
(213) 991-6302

Stainless Medical Products (The Wildcat)
9389 Dowdy Dr.
San Diego, Ca., 92126
(800) 238-6678

REFERENCES:

1) *Accent on Living* is published quarterly. It costs $6.00 per year. To subscribe, write: P. O. Box 700, Bloomington, Ill. 61701.

2) Gottschalk, B.; Sarette, M.: Three Wheeled Scooters: How to Choose the Best for You. *Accent on Living* Vol. 29:2 (Fall) Pages 32—38, 1984.

3) *Paraplegia News*. 5201 North 19th Ave., Suite 111, Phoenix, AZ, 85015. Published monthly. Price $12.00 per year.

Chapter 3

Wheelchair Access
A Privilege You Deserve

By Steven N. Fellows

There is an old stereotype that disability means you can't take care of yourself. Avoid that idea. It imprisons body and mind. This chapter is about *moving*—safely— around your home and your community.

The transition from walking erect without physical impairment, to walking with great difficulty or moving only on wheels, is the source of much of the horror of MS. MSers have to cope with this possibility. But if you approach these changes as a series of lesser problems to be solved one by one, you will cope more successfully.

Early in my disease, I was convinced that I must accept a short, unhappy life of being pushed around in a wheelchair by an attendant. It has been ten years since my diagnosis. I do need a wheelchair, but I roll *myself* up and down ramps and curb cuts, into banks, stores, churches and government buildings. When I want to go home, I roll to my car, which I have parked in a convenient handicapped parking space. There I load myself and my chair into the car, and drive home. Once home, I roll into the house, and roll wherever I wish. I chase the kids, take a shower, raid the refrigerator and go to my shop, where I make many messes and occasional pieces of furniture. I have access to my world.

THE LAW

Congress passed the 1973 Rehabilitation Act with little public reaction. This law contains section 504, a single paragraph that prohibits discrimination against people because they are disabled. Section 504 has become a most significant piece of federal legislation.

Thirty-two federal agencies were instructed to write specific regulations that prevent federally funded agencies from discriminating against disabled clients. Basically, the regulations warned: "If you discriminate against disabled people, you will lose federal funding."

By mid-1977, when none of the federal agencies had actually written "504" regulations, disabled activists staged a hunger strike at the Department of Health, Education and Welfare, HEW (now the Department of Health and Human Services, HHS). This display forced HEW officials to act. Now disabled people have the right to demand that the federal government withhold money from recipients who fail to provide access to their clients. As a result, local and state governments, educational institutions, and other recipients of federal funds have modified their programs and their buildings.

"504" regulations are useful, but because their meaning may still be unclear, they have not become a legal panacea for all access ills. For instance, recipients of federal funds and disabled advocates may interpret a phrase like "reasonable access" quite differently. Enforcement is cumbersome, and may require intervention by federal officials. Last, expensive federal regulations become a target for political manipulation.

Nonetheless, "504" regulations have survived the transition from a liberal administration to a conservative one. The Office of Revenue Sharing, an important distributor of federal funds, recently promulgated "504" regulations despite strong conservative pressure to return government control to the states.

Section 504 and its many regulations have helped to educate architects, urban planners, politicians and, perhaps most important of all, the courts. The following true story illustrates how "504" can work.

Our courthouse in Tompkins County, N.Y., was inaccessible, and the county administration had no intention of remodeling. Local disabled advocates decided against invoking "504." Instead, they sued the county using New York State's "sunshine law." This law requires that public meetings be accessible to the public. The case came to trial in less than a month. In less than 20 minutes, the judge ordered the county to hold all meetings in an accessible place.

In order to reach his decision, the judge had to define access. Many meetings were routinely held on the second floor of a building with no elevator and no ground level entrance. A mobility impaired person could be carried upstairs to a meeting, but the judge said "No!" Had this case been tried before passage of "504," and before people started thinking about the meaning of access, the judge might easily have decided in favor of the county.

County meetings were moved to a more accessible but less comfortable place. County officials soon chose to return to the plush chairs and paneled walls they had formerly enjoyed. As a result, our courthouse has a ramped entrance, accessible bathrooms, an elevator and raised signs for the visually impaired. Only the naïve can believe that access solutions will always be as simple as my courthouse example, but we cannot deny that things are improving. Interestingly, county taxpayers seem happy about the outcome of this saga.

ACCESS TO YOUR HOME

During most of this chapter, we shall discuss ideas to make your home more accessible. Unfortunately, every suggestion costs money. You cannot afford to make every possible modification. Use this chapter as a beginning resource, perhaps as a check list, certainly not as a Bible.

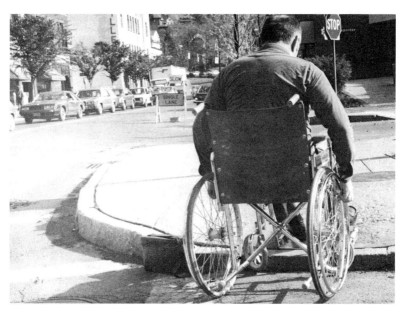

Fig. 3-1. Faulty curb cut whose lip is almost as high as the front wheels!

Planning to Build or Remodel

Before you plan your new home or your remodeling job, make a list of everything that irritates you in your present home, and all the things that might irritate you

if you were more disabled. MSers know they may
sometime need an electric wheelchair or a full time
attendant. Prepare for the worst. Be totally pessimistic
about the future course of your disease. I bought a split
level home in 1977, thinking the stairs would provide
me an incentive to exercise. At the time, I walked with
a cane, but just four years later I spent a lot more money
to make the house wheelchair accessible. There is no

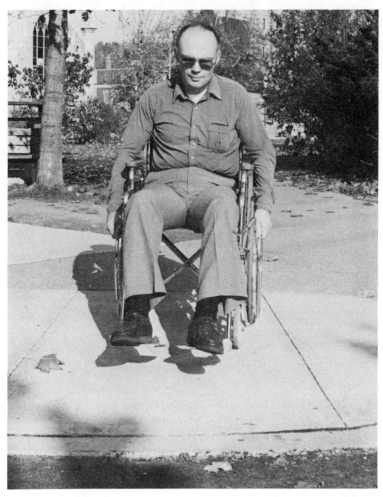

**Fig. 3-2. Perfectly constructed curb cut, with no
lip at base of ramp.**

value in buying, building or remodeling, if you have to do it all over again just four years later!

Talk to other disabled people who have modified their homes. Collect ideas from accessible public places, but expect to find mistakes there, too. One of our local department stores installed accessible bathrooms. The men's room contained a well designed toilet stall with proper railings and a door that opened out. There was also a special sink with an extended lip and "quad" lever faucet handles, but the sink had been installed in *front* of the toilet stall, leaving only 21 inches of clearance. A wheelchair requires a minimum of 27 inches to squeak through. The wheeler could wash his hands in style, but could never use that toilet stall!

Even the vast supply of "expert" planners, architects and engineers from the federal government make mistakes. Curb cuts with three inch lips are not uncommon (Fig. 3-1). Learn from mistakes, and applaud well done projects (Fig. 3-2).

Specifications and Resources

MSers must design their homes with an eye to money as well as individual need. At least there is no shortage of design ideas. Hospital rehabilitation units, occupational therapy and prosthetics departments (especially from Veteran's Administration hospitals), local advocate organizations and national organizations, such as the MS and Easter Seal Societies are all potential sources of information.

Libraries usually have literature about access. Ask the librarian for help in finding them. Be certain the information is recent. New ideas surface every year.

Several magazines contain up-to-date information about products not mentioned in catalogs and other

Fig. 3-3. Graphic Conventions.

Graphic Conventions

Convention	Description
36 / 915 (dimension line)	Typical dimension line showing U.S. customary units (in inches) above the line and SI units (in millimeters) below
9 / 230 (on extended line)	Dimensions for short distances indicated on extended line
9 / 230, 36 / 915	Dimension line showing alternate dimensions required
(arrow)	Direction of approach
max	Maximum
min	Minimum
(dotted line)	Boundary of clear floor area
℄	Centerline

standard sources. *Accent on Living* (1)* and *Paraplegia News* (2)* have answers to many of your questions about elevators, hand controls and other mobility aids.

---

* Note: Addresses for this literature may be found on page 79.

Section 504 regulations demanded that public buildings be accessible, but provided no consistent definition of "accessible." Clear architectural standards were needed. The American National Standard, *Specifications for Making Buildings and Facilities Accessible to and Usable by Physically Handicapped People*, ANSI A117.1, 1980 (3) is the result of five years of research conducted at Syracuse University. Disabled advocates welcomed the new publication because it ensured that Standard architectural provisions would meet their needs. The 1980 Standard is still deficient in some respects, so we can expect another revision in the next few years. Even so, the 1980 Standard is a most useful aid in designing accessible buildings.

A few figures from the 1980 ANSI Standard are included in this chapter. These figures would be difficult to understand without Fig. 3-3, the Table of Conventions, which explains how to read the rest of the figures.

To the uninitiated, the Standard appears to demand excessive space, but people who depend on crutches, walkers and wheelchairs have a different perspective from those who walk. When the uninitiated ignore the Standard, the result is unwarranted expense for things that do not work!

Wheelchairs, whether operated by passenger or attendant, cannot be turned on a dime, and cannot be backed up unless there is room for the front wheels to turn around on their casters. Elbows and knuckles add to the effective width of a wheelchair. Toes add to its length. A wheelchair is exceedingly rough on furniture, trim, protruding walls, corners, baseboards, pets and people. The wheels and footrests seem to seek out things to attack. There is no cure for the rambunctious wheel-

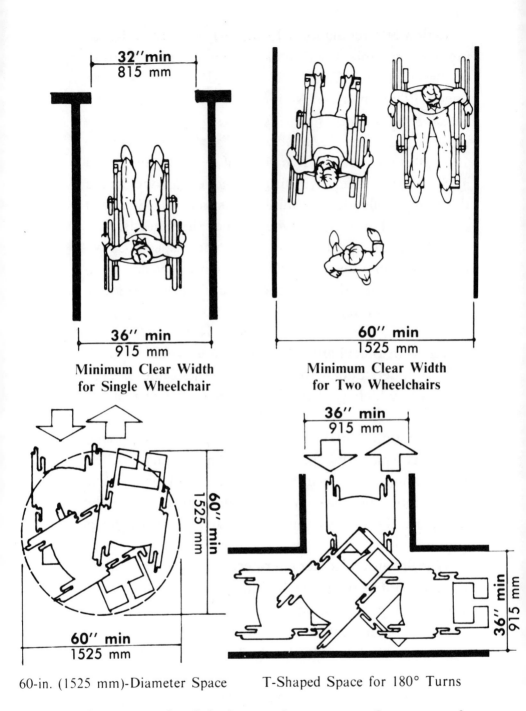

32" min
815 mm

36" min
915 mm

Minimum Clear Width
for Single Wheelchair

60" min
1525 mm

Minimum Clear Width
for Two Wheelchairs

60" min
1525 mm

60" min
1525 mm

60-in. (1525 mm)-Diameter Space

36" min
915 mm

36" min
915 mm

T-Shaped Space for 180° Turns

**Fig. 3-4. Wheelchair turning spaces. Courtesy of
the American National Standards Institute.**

chair, but adequate maneuvering space helps to prevent it from terrorizing the family and destroying the house.

Fig. 3-4 illustrates some of the dimensions required for maneuvering a loaded chair. A five foot diameter is *required* to turn the chair around without resorting to an automobile style "Y" turn.

Economic Considerations

Building and remodeling costs go far beyond the price of construction. Additional space requires more housework. Remodeling often results in higher property taxes, larger heating and cooling bills, greater insurance costs and added maintenance. Keep all of these in mind as you make your plans. If you are building or remodeling to meet medical needs, you may qualify for income tax rebates and property tax reductions. Contact your local assessment office about local property tax rules.

Careful planning can lessen utility bills and housework. Plan floor spaces to minimize travel distances between household chores. Study floor plans in magazines, in contractor's offices and lumber yards. Contact your local power company and reliable building contractors while you design spaces and plan insulation. Look at adapted homes in your community. Learn from mistakes other people have already made. Use their successful solutions in your own plans. Ask lots of questions first! *Then* pick up hammer and saw.

Think Positively

My accessible home is not a nursing home. Yours need not be either, no matter how severe your disability. My kids roll their "Big Wheels" down the driveway, into the garage, up the ramp into the kitchen, through the house to the front door and down the sidewalk to the driveway, just as I do. They understand that access works for them, too.

Getting in the Door

The dirtiest four letter word in my vocabulary is *step*. But steps may be conquered by various methods, depending on physical impairment, availability of space, and of course, money.

For the walking disabled who drag their toes, steps can be built without a projecting overhang at little cost. This is only a temporary solution for most MSers, because several years in the future, the walking MSer may need wheelchair access. Homes are seldom built with entrances at ground level, but ramps and elevators are good solutions for most situations.

Ramps

Ramps are better than elevators in many situations. They have no moving parts and require no electricity. They are relatively inexpensive to build, and require no regular maintenance.

A ramp should never exceed a rise-over-run ratio of 1:12, and should have a less steep rise if possible (Fig. 3-5). You may be aware of the formula, but not know why it is important. Steep ramps are dangerous. Many of us can *climb* a steeper ramp, but we cannot keep a wheelchair from tipping over backward as we do! Do not let anyone talk you into building a steeper, cheaper, and therefore more dangerous ramp, unless there is absolutely no alternative and you will have an attendant every time you climb it.

Ramps should be at least 36 inches wide. Install hand rails on each side. Railings provide an alternative way to

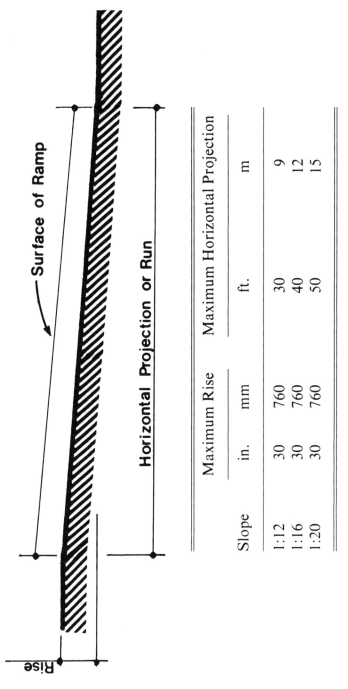

Slope	Maximum Rise		Maximum Horizontal Projection	
	in.	mm	ft.	m
1:12	30	760	30	9
1:16	30	760	40	12
1:20	30	760	50	15

Fig. 3-5. Sample ramp dimensions. Courtesy of the American National Standards Institute.

climb and descend without having to grip those skinny little wheel rims that seemed just the right size on the level. Railings are usually installed 32 to 36 inches above the ramp surface. People of average height usually like their railings installed at 35 to 36 inches. If you are short, consider installing your railings lower. Get a tape measure and check the heights of railings in your community to decide for yourself.

The railings themselves should be $1^{1}/_{4}$ to $1^{1}/_{2}$ inches in diameter for an easy grip, and should have $1^{1}/_{2}$ inches clearance from walls, to prevent skinned knuckles. Specifications for the height, diameter and clearance of railings are critical for good grip and safety (Fig. 3-6). If you can't easily get your hands around them and hang on, they lose their value.

Most wheelers can climb a 30 foot run comfortably without a rest. After every thirty feet, plan to have a level section five feet long. This will ensure that front and back wheels are off the incline while you rest. Remember also to design a level space in front of the door.

Elevator

Ramps may not work in buildings with limited interior or exterior spaces, nor for wheelers with weak arms. At least four different kinds of elevator are available. The Stair Glide® is a simple seat that rides up and down stairs on a rail (Fig. 3-7). The Stair Glide does not carry wheelchairs, and is unsafe for people with poor balance. It does not work outside. The Stair Glide is less expensive than most other elevators, and is quite popular because it is adaptable to many interior designs.

The Porch Lift® is a vertical elevator for use inside or

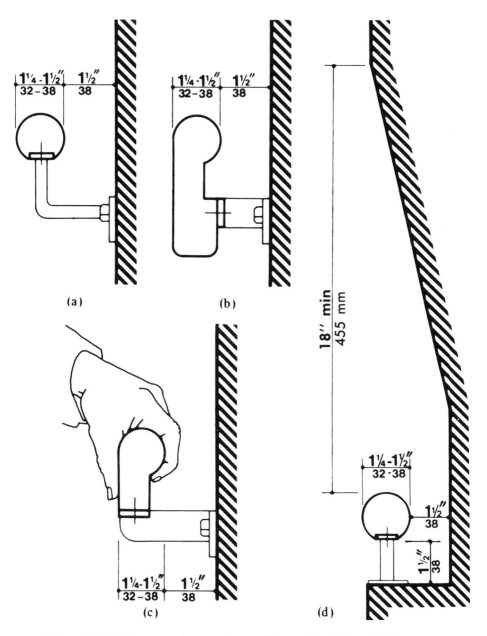

Fig. 3-6. Size and spacing of hand rail grab bars. Courtesy of the American National Standards Institute.

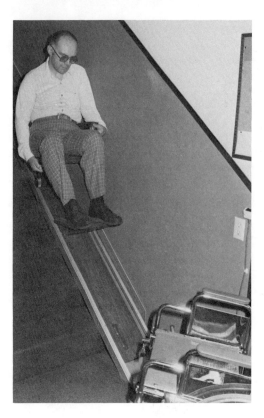

Fig. 3-7. The Stair glide, by American Stair Glide Corp, Grandview, MO. 64030. Photograph courtesy of the Ellis Hollow Apartments, Ithaca, N.Y.

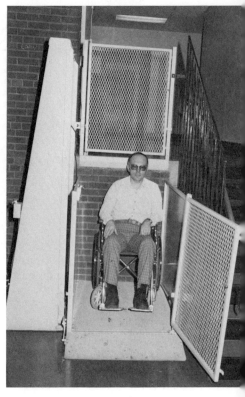

Fig. 3-8. The Porch Lift, also by American Stair Glide Corp. Photograph courtesy of the Greater Ithaca Activities Center, Ithaca, N.Y.

outdoors (Fig. 3-8). Once a Porch Lift is installed in a narrow stairwell, the stairs may be lost to normal traffic.

The Butler Chair Lift carries a wheelchair, a person seated in a simple chair, or a person standing (Fig. 3-9). When it is parked at the bottom of the stairs, pedestrians simply walk over it and up the stairs.

Built-in elevators are nice, but they are expensive. If you install a built-in elevator, be sure it is large enough for your needs now, and in the future.

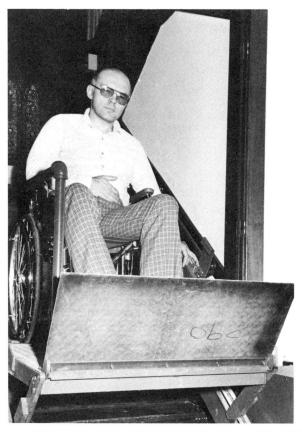

Fig. 3-9. The Butler Chair Lift, by Flinchbaugh Corporation, 390 Eberts Lane, York, PA. 17403. Photograph courtesy of St. John's Episcopal Church, Ithaca, N.Y.

Doors

Doors can become major obstructions. Users of Canadian crutches remember when someone kindly tried to "help" by opening the door after the crutcher had shifted weight in order to grab the door knob. The resulting loss of balance is unforgettable. Doors are even harder for wheelers to use.

Problems start in front of the door, where the wheelchair must be stable while the wheeler unlocks and opens the door. If the door swings toward the wheeler, it must clear the chair. Once through, space is needed to maneuver the chair and close the door.

The 1980 ANSI Standard shows the dimensions needed for almost any imaginable approach to a hinged door. (Fig.3-10). Study this figure carefully as you plan.

Door knobs are a problem for MSers with poor grip. Blade, or "quad" handles are a good and easy way to ease frustration (Fig. 3-11). Adhesive tape wrapped around door knobs isn't pretty, but it makes them easier to turn.

Pneumatic door openers allow the hurrying wheeler or the tired crutcher to move right through without worry about bugs and burglars, and they usually can be adjusted to any desired pressure.

Examine Fig. 3-12 carefully. It illustrates the necessary "clear opening" of several kinds of doorway. A 34 inch doorway shrinks to 32 inches *or less* when a hinged door is opened. Wheelers can use arms and elbows to squeeze through a clear opening of about 27 inches, but this scrapes trim, door, fingers and chair. Aim for 32 inches or more with the door open.

Garage doors are trouble. It is impossible to open a garage door from a wheelchair while sitting outside on a patch of ice during a miserable winter's night. Auto-

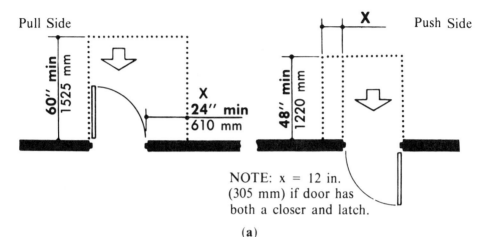

Pull Side

60″ min 1525 mm

X
24″ min
610 mm

Push Side

X

48″ min 1220 mm

NOTE: x = 12 in.
(305 mm) if door has
both a closer and latch.

(**a**)
Front Approaches — Swinging Doors

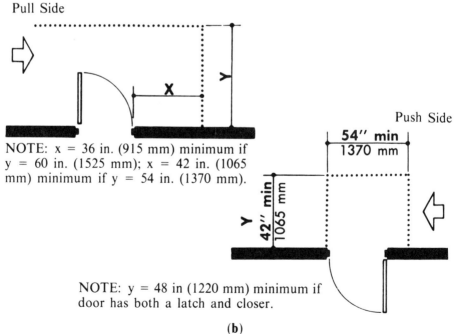

Pull Side

X

Y

NOTE: x = 36 in. (915 mm) minimum if
y = 60 in. (1525 mm); x = 42 in. (1065
mm) minimum if y = 54 in. (1370 mm).

Push Side

54″ min
1370 mm

Y
42″ min 1065 mm

NOTE: y = 48 in (1220 mm) minimum if
door has both a latch and closer.

(**b**)
Hinge Side Approaches — Swinging Doors

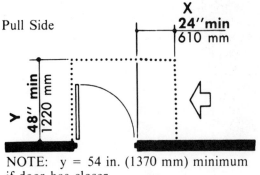

Pull Side

X
24"min
610 mm

Y
48" min
1220 mm

NOTE: y = 54 in. (1370 mm) minimum
if door has closer.

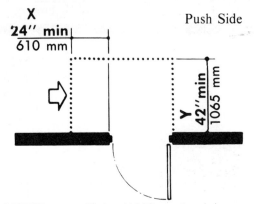

Push Side

X
24" min
610 mm

Y
42"min
1065 mm

NOTE: y =48 in. (1220 mm) minimum
if door has closer.

(c)
Latch Side Approaches — Swinging Doors

NOTE: All doors in alcoves shall comply with the clearances
for front approaches.

Fig. 3-10. Maneuvering clearances at doors. Courtesy of the American National Standards Institute.

matic door openers do it all from inside the car or garage. They are relatively easy for any able bodied, reasonably intelligent person to install. Start dropping strong birthday hints!

Patio and pocket doors are easy to open and close. They do not protrude into the maneuvering space. Patio

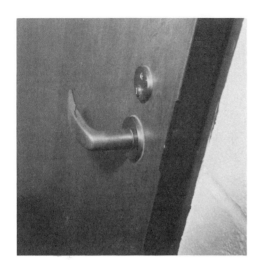

Fig. 3-11. Blade, or "quad" door handle. Photograph courtesy of the Greater Ithaca Activities Center, Ithaca, N.Y.

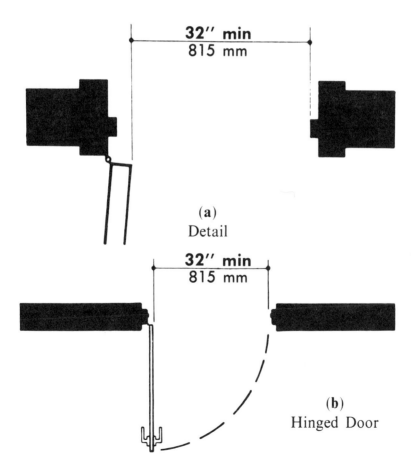

32" min
815 mm

(a)
Detail

32" min
815 mm

(b)
Hinged Door

doors have tracks along the bottom that hinder easy wheeling and walking, while pocket doors (Fig. 3-12c) hang from an overhead track. Because there is no track at the base of a pocket door, it does not seal out wind and rain as patio doors do, so it cannot be used as an outside door. It is excellent as an inside door because it is always out of the way.

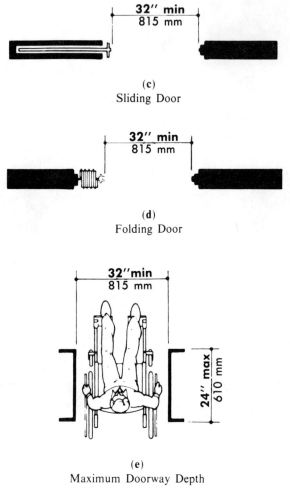

(c)
Sliding Door

(d)
Folding Door

(e)
Maximum Doorway Depth

Fig. 3-12. Accessible doorway dimensions. Courtesy of the American National Standards Institute.

Kitchens

Kitchens may be the center of family life, as well as the place to prepare food. Even if the wheeler is not the family cook, many meals will be eaten in the kitchen. So plan spaces to accommodate the entire family. ANSI's weakest area for home owners is the kitchen.

Ranges

The range should have a roll in space 30 inches wide, at least 19 inches deep (front to back), with at least 27 inches of knee clearance from the floor, so a wheeler can sit comfortably to cook. If the top is 32 to 34 inches from the floor, cooking remains comfortable for wheelers or anyone else who likes to sit while stirring the soup.

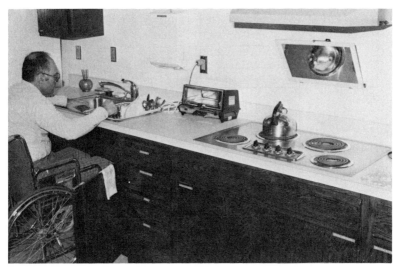

Fig. 3-13. Accessible kitchen sink and range. Photograph courtesy of the Tompkins County Community Hospital, Ithaca, N.Y.

Burners arranged in a semicircle, with up front controls (Fig. 3-13) allow easy control of cooking temperatures without reaching across hot burners and cookware. Note the mirror above the range, which is adjusted to show the seated chef what is going on inside pots and pans.

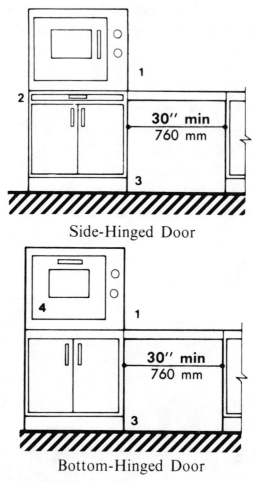

Side-Hinged Door

Bottom-Hinged Door

SYMBOL KEY:
1. Countertop or wall-mounted oven.
2. Pull-out board preferred with side-opening door.
3. Clear open space.
4. Bottom-hinged door.

Fig. 3-14. Counter top dimensions and oven door options. Courtesy of the American National Standards Institute.

Ovens

Wall mounted conventional or microwave ovens place food at a height where the chef need not bend precariously to put pans in, baste food, or inspect the progress of cooking. Wall mounted ovens come with side opening and down swinging doors (Fig. 3-14). Wheelers usually like the side swinging doors. They swing out of the way when we roll close to the oven. A shelf under the door helps to support heavy, hot dishes.

Refrigerator

Side by side refrigerator-freezer combinations are said to be best for wheelers, but your author's waistline provides mute testimony that ice cream stacked on top is still accessible. Stacked refrigerator-freezer combinations should have doors that can be changed to open either to the left or right. The individual can choose the easiest installation.

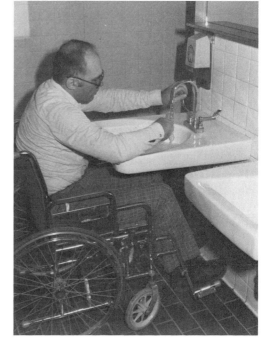

Fig. 3-15. Accessible sink with blade or "quad" faucets. Photograph courtesy of the Center Ithaca Building, Ithaca, New York.

Sinks

Sinks should have the same roll in capacity as the range. Shop carefully for faucets. Blade, or "quad" faucets are usually found in handicapped accessible bathrooms (Fig. 3-15). Delta® single lever faucets are popular in many homes and are excellent for those with disability of one or both arms (Fig. 3-16). If you prefer a large knob, get the Delta type faucet with knob instead of lever.

Place water and drain lines as close to the wall as possible. Insulate hot water pipes to prevent burns on legs and feet.

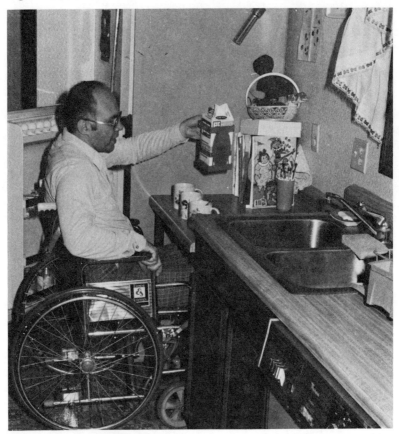

Fig. 3-16. Roll-in work counter. Kitchen sink has a Delta® faucet.

Tables

Never bring a table home from the store until you have rolled yourself comfortably under it. Low table underpinnings discriminate against wheelchairs. Unhappy is the wheeler who sits far back from dinner!

On the other hand, Virginia Hedrick, of Visalia, California, reports that opened kitchen drawers, topped with trays, make excellent tables for herself and her wheeler husband. They save carrying food from stove to dining room, too!

Cabinets and Storage Spaces

Cooking habits and family size determine how much accessible storage space and cooking space you need. There is no perfect solution. Any design must be based on the position of appliances and furniture.

As you plan your wheelchair accessible kitchen, consider one more problem. Wheelers want roll in work surfaces. They also want under counter storage space that can be reached from a sitting position. Obviously, the old adage applies here. You can't have your accessible counter and store things under it.

Think about these things too:

Drawers and lazy Susans work well. With a slight push or pull, everything in them is accessible.

Built-in pantries with dozens of shelves mounted on doors and inside swinging units are excellent storage spaces for wheelers (Fig. 3-17).

Under the counter cupboards with handles mounted at the top of the door and large roll out bins provide accessible storage. Don't forget to leave space for the wheelchair! If you install cupboards above the counter, mount the handles at the bottom of the doors.

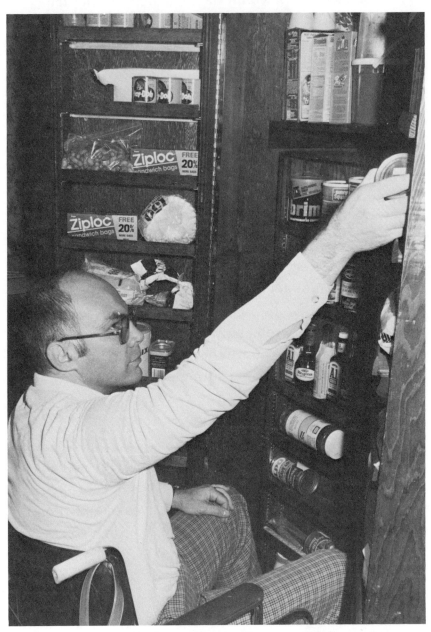

Fig. 3-17. Built-in pantry. Two swing-out doors
provide 42 wheelchair accessible shelves.

Mechanical grabbers allow wheelers to reach at least the lower shelves of high cupboards, while reserving upper shelves for dead storage. They do not work well for heavy objects, though. Beware the bottle of vinegar in the grabber. If hands are weak and incoordinated, it may drop suddenly into your lap—or onto your head!

Work Counters

When we remodeled, I designed one short length of roll in work counter (Fig. 3-16) at 32 inches above the floor. It has a 29 inch knee clearance. The opening is 30 inches wide and 24 inches deep. A cooking wheeler may want more space.

I have never been able to use that counter. The kids got there first with their crayons, paints, books and a stool. They know accessible work space when they see it! It is fine with me, though. I never did like to peel potatoes. The counter keeps the kids out from under my wheels while we are in the kitchen together!

Bathrooms

Bathroom access begins at the entrance to the house. You need an unobstructed path from the door, directly to the bathroom: no stairs, no furniture in the way, no narrow, cramped hallways or clumsy doors. Once arrived, you need enough space in the bathroom to maneuver easily. Of all the rooms in the house, the bathroom requires most planning. The constant frustration of a minimally accessible bathroom is heightened in times of emergency. MSers have injured themselves in unsafe and poorly planned bathrooms.

As you design your bathroom, draw some full scale floor plans with chalk on the surface of an open space, like the driveway or garage floor. Try it out before you

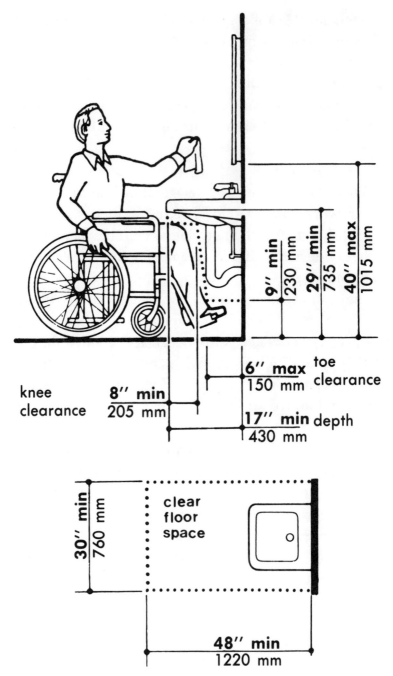

9" min
230 mm

29" min
735 mm

40" max
1015 mm

6" max   toe
150 mm   clearance

knee
clearance

8" min
205 mm

17" min depth
430 mm

30" min
760 mm

clear
floor
space

48" min
1220 mm

Fig. 3-19. Lavatory dimensions (top), and clear floor space for sinks. Courtesy of the American National Standards Institute.

build. Don't discover too late that you made some subtle but expensive mistake.

Bathroom Sinks

Use the same guidelines for installation of bathroom and kitchen sinks. Consider whether the advantages of a sink with an extended lip are outweighed by its clumsy appearance (Fig. 3-15). Examine the ANSI Standard measurements for sink, medicine cabinet and maneuvering space (Fig. 3-18).

A roll in sink eliminates the traditional under sink vanity, but bathroom scales and cleaning supplies store nicely in a small closet in the bathroom. Be certain the route to the closet is accessible when the door is open.

Medicine Cabinets and Mirrors

If there are no small children in the house, mount the medicine cabinet with its base 40 inches off the floor or lower. Cabinets with built-in tilted mirrors are available and convenient for the wheeler. If there are small children, get a lock for the door.

A single medicine cabinet cannot be installed to serve the whole family. When the cabinet is mounted at the usual height, only the bottom shelf is readily accessible to the wheeler, the second shelf with fingertips, and the third might as well be Mount Everest. If the mirror is also mounted in the conventional vertical manner, the wheeler can see only a hair-do. If the conventional height cabinet is fitted with a tilted mirror, the wheeler still cannot reach top shelves, while the rest of the family have fine views of their navels!

Install two medicine cabinets if you have the money and space, so people of all heights have storage space and mirrors that work. If space is limited, install a mirror flush with the wall above the sink for standing members, and the medicine cabinet lower. The wheeler has visibility, and everyone has accessible storage. Don't forget the lock!

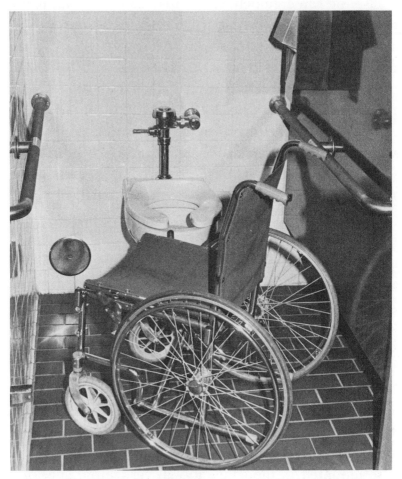

Fig. 3-19. Raised toilet seat eases transfers. Photograph courtesy of the Center Ithaca Building, Ithaca, N.Y.

Toilets

Accessible public toilets are different from the ones at home. Public stalls have toilet seats raised about three inches higher than the conventional toilet, to help people stand up from a seated position, and to help wheelers transfer directly from the wheelchair to the toilet. Fig. 3-19 illustrates a raised toilet seat level with the wheelchair seat. Fig. 3-20 illustrates a wheelchair parked next to a conventional toilet. As you plan, consider the raised toilet seats for possible use at home and check the placement of grab bars at the same time.

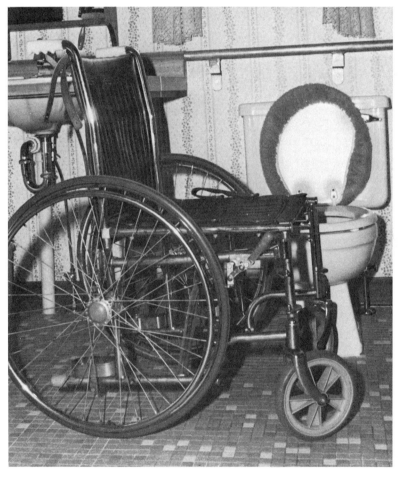

Fig. 3-20. Transfer from standard height toilet is more difficult. Inexpensive inserts are available to raise this seat to wheelchair height.

If you want a cheaper solution, consider buying an inexpensive toilet insert at your Physician's and Hospital Supply store, which can be removed for cleaning. Some inserts may be set at any height you like best.

Placement of bathroom grab bars and railings is a matter of personal preference. The 1980 ANSI Standard illustrates several alternative systems, and even illustrates two different transfer methods to show how the systems work. I was privileged to examine plans for a housing project that included several accessible apartments. Bathroom arrangements were identical in all apartments and looked well planned to me, but when I invited another wheeler to look at the plans, he declared he could not possibly transfer to the toilet!

Use the ANSI Standard to determine the height, diameter and length of grab bars, and their distance from the walls. Do not let anyone tell you where to place the railings. You know best! A safe bathroom for me, might be the cause of a wrenched back or broken hip for you.

Bathing

Bathing is often frustrating and dangerous, even for ambulatory MSers. Many of us know the horror of discovering we have no strength to get out of the tub after a wonderful hot bath. As the disease progresses, the bathtub becomes a place of daily struggle: getting in or out over the side, or falling frequently. Because of the tub, some MSers give up private bathing.

Simple Solutions

The hot soak may be a luxury of the past, but you can still bathe alone until disability becomes extremely severe. If you have no alternative to the tub, a bathtub seat and proper railings are a standard and relatively inexpensive solution. The ANSI Standard provides some guidance here, but the best way to decide is to find other people with adapted bathrooms. Perhaps they will let you take a bath in their tub, or at least try transferring in and out of it.

The bather must be able to transfer to the tub seat and move independently into position for showering. MSers with poor balance find this method disagreeable unless there is additional support on the seat. They need one hand to hold on with, while the other does the washing.

Hand held, detachable shower heads with water hoses about five feet long are an advantage. They allow a bather to spray parts of the body that might not be accessible from a fixed source. Detachable sprays are mounted on a vertical pole so they can be raised and lowered to serve a seated or standing bather.

Roll-in Shower

If you can afford it, a roll-in shower is the best solution of all. Be sure your plans include enough space in the shower for an attendant plus you and the shower chair. Drainage must be adequate to ensure that the water does not escape into the bathroom, but even a low curb should be avoided.

> "We solved the drainage problem by lowering the shower room floor 1 1/2 inches. We then built a wooden slat floor flush with the rest of the room." wrote one of our editors, when he read this section. "The wooden floor can be removed for cleaning. It is comfortable to stand on when it's cold, and because we used cedar floor boards, there are no splinters."

Place a continuous railing around the inside of the shower for everyone's safety. Chairs slide, even with the wheels locked, and wheels spin easily on wet surfaces. Railings help you to control these problems.

One last thing about your roll-in shower: You will have to fight the rest of the family to use it. They will all love it and consider it their personal property.

Controls and Shower Heads

Shower faucets are usually a single "quad" lever or knob. Examine available styles to determine which you like best. Buy a temperature sensing control valve to prevent burns from a sudden increase in water temperature when someone flushes the toilet in the basement, or freezing chills when the dishwasher comes on in the kitchen.

Miscellaneous Considerations

Switches and Outlets

MSers are at a disadvantage when they have to stoop or bend to reach wall outlets at baseboard level. It is awkward to reach across a counter from a wheelchair for switches or electrical and telephone connections. You can move those switches, plugs thermostats and rheostats. When you do, have them relocated 18 to 48 inches above the floor, where they are handy. Put them on the front of cupboards and under counters in the kitchen, where they will be easy to reach.

Floors

Proper rugs improve mobility for crutchers and wheelers. Luxurious pile rugs catch at dragging feet and cause tremendous resistance even against thin, non-pneumatic wheelchair tires. Low pile industrial carpet reduces these problems. But even low pile carpets cause some drag. I chose bare wood and tile floors. Their slippery surfaces were more dangerous when I walked with crutch or cane, but they allow my wheelchair free passage. If you choose tile, avoid rough surfaced material. It is hard to clean, and the vibration on the wheels causes leg and bladder spasms.

Halls

Design your hallways as short and as wide (at least 40 inches) as possible. Keep them free of furniture. Wheelchairs do not move precisely. In times of urgency, they bump into walls, baseboards and people. Eliminate hallways if you can, but if you cannot, make them wide enough for easy travel.

Closet Rods and Hooks

Standard hanger rods and hooks are installed 66 inches from the floor. The ANSI Standard recommends 54 inches for wheelchair access, but this leaves some clothes dragging on the floor. Get someone to hold clothes on hangers at different heights, while you practice reaching. You may decide to leave some hangers high to keep dresses off the floor, and place others lower for convenience.

TRANSPORTATION

Public Transportation

In the first edition of this book, I began this section by writing: "Public transportation will be truly public when disabled people have as much access to it as the rest of the public." The United States Department of Public Transportation had originally issued "504" regulations, and then withdrawn them for re-evaluation. As we prepare this volume, the Department is still working on the problem and trying to enforce interim regulations. The trouble is the same now as it was before: imperfect technology and fixed, wrong attitudes about disability.

Technology is a major problem. The kneeling bus is a useful modification and has a good record for reliability, but the shallow steps for cane and crutch users help only some disabled people. Mechanical lifts for wheelchairs have a poor maintenance record, so transportation companies avoid them.

Problems of attitude are equally difficult. Bus drivers and administrators often believe that public transportation can't work for disabled people. They make little effort to encourage use of their services. Most public transportation systems rely on small busses or vans to provide door to door service. There is no fixed schedule, so the disabled, unlike the able, must wait a day or a week to go shopping.

It's even worse in bad weather. The ice and snow of northern winters is so treacherous that many disabled people stay home, even if transportation *is* available.

For those who can afford it, and have the necessary coordination of arms and hands, modified transportation is available and effective. Unhappily, these modifications are beyond the means of many disabled people.

Driving

Aids for a wide range of physical disability enable disabled people to drive safely and comfortably. Magazines like *Paraplegia News* are filled with advertisements for simple hand controls and other vehicle control systems. Their complexity is limited only by your financial resources. It is essential to have your system installed by an expert. Veterans Administration Hospital prosthetics departments usually have information about equipment and installation.

Hand Controls

Basic hand controls drive the vehicle without using feet. They allow use of foot pedals by physically healthy drivers. Usually there is a single gas/brake lever and a spinner knob (Fig. 3-21), or a spoked "quad" grip for steering with one hand.

Gas/brake combinations work in one of two ways. In both designs, the lever hangs under the steering wheel and protrudes to the left or right, depending on preference. In both systems, brakes are applied by pushing forward on the lever. With the simpler control, the lever is pulled back to accelerate. This allows either gas *or* brake to be applied, but not both.

The mechanics of the second system are slightly more complex. Push the lever forward to brake, but pull it down, toward the thigh, to accelerate. This system allows the driver to apply gas and brake at the same time, a handy feature if you have stopped for a light on a hill. This second system must be adjusted carefully, or the lever may hit the driver's thigh before the accelerator is fully depressed. Most hand controls can be purchased and installed for around $700.

Gas/brake levers mounted on the left side of the steering column are dangerous if they strike the window crank. Imagine your horror when you push the lever to brake, it hits the window crank, and nothing happens! This possibility prompted me to buy power windows for my hand controlled automobile. The power windows and power locks provide better ventilation and better security.

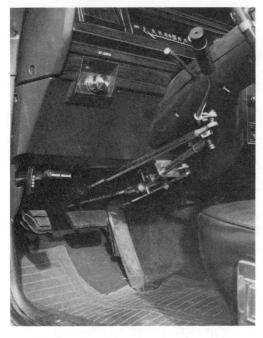

Fig. 3-21. Hand controls. Spinner knob on the steering wheel is on the opposite side from hand controls while driving. Gas/brake lever, turn signals, horn and dimmer switch are all easily accessible to the left hand.

Buttons and Switches

Do you drive at night using only low beams because you cannot reach the foot dimmer switch? There are at least two remedies. New cars often come with the dimmer switch mounted on the turn signal arm. If yours does not, you can mount a hand operated dimmer switch on the hand control lever. Install a horn control button next to it for convenience.

Turn signal, windshield wipers, dimmer and horn are usually mounted on the left side of the steering column. If you mount your gas/brake lever on the right and steer with the left hand, you can transfer the other functions to the right as well, using extender levers.

Seats

The wrong seat leaves the driver cramped, crowded, out of reach of the controls, blind to surroundings and unsupported. This is a disaster for MSers with poor balance. Disabled drivers prefer power seats for better comfort and safety. I tried several types before I bought reclining split bench seats with arm rests.

Swivel seats make it easier to get in and out of the car, but you must be able to turn the seat unassisted. Swivel seats are especially useful for passenger MSers if an attendant must help with transfers.

Additional Equipment

Air conditioning is a great advantage for heat-sensitive MSers. It allows the MSer to arrive rested and fresh after a summer drive.

Cruise control relieves the driver from constant attention to the hand controls. It frees one hand to do other things.

Remote controlled right-hand mirrors help with backing and passing.

Tilt-steering wheels provide more room to get in and out of the car. Some drivers tilt the wheel as they drive to relieve arm and shoulder strain.

Choosing a Vehicle

No one can choose your car for you. Talk to other MSers, paraplegics, amputees. Ask to sit in their cars. Try the controls. Load your crutches or wheelchair into the car. Listen to their ideas and complaints. Some disabled people stay with the same car and controls for years. Others try something different every time they trade.

Many wheelers choose large two door sedans because they can slip the wheelchair behind the front seat after they get in. After many transfers, upholstery suffers from this practice. I chose a large station wagon with roof rack. I can still shuffle a short distance with support, so I load the chair in the back, grab onto the roof rack, and shuffle forward to the driver's seat. This leaves more room for my family in the back seat, and keeps the chair safely inside the car.

Vans with power lifts are ever so nice—and ever so expensive! Some are designed so the wheeler never leaves the wheelchair, but drives seated in it. The lift won't work with a dead battery, and the engine may not start if the battery is weakened from many loadings. If you buy such a vehicle, insist on a two battery system for more reserve power.

The Terrible Cost of Transportation

Some states require power steering and automatic transmission for hand controlled cars. A large car with extra power equipment gets poor mileage, and is more expensive to buy and maintain than a stripped-down compact, but it does provide independence and a comfortable ride to work.

If you buy car and equipment especially to compensate for your medical condition, your physician can write a prescription for it. This will probably earn you a tax rebate next April. Consult a government pamphlet on medical and disability tax deductions, or talk to a tax consultant as you prepare your return.

You may despair of owning such a luxury liner. Many disabled people drive a second hand car with just enough equipment to keep them on the road. They complain, but they remain independent!

> "We're frantically trying to get ready for a trip to the Grand Canyon (Frantic and MS do not mix!!)," wrote Bonnie Johannes, of Great Falls, Montana. "Somewhere along the course of this disease, the words *stubbornness* and *ingenuity* come into play. Fortunately, my husband is mechanically inclined and I am a seamstress and creative. Between the two of us, we usually solve problems without spending a lot of money or going to an orthopedic supply house.
>
> "My hand controls came from Mobility Products and Design, inc., 709 Kentucky St., Vallejo, CA, 94590. It was already fitted with horn and dimmer switch, and my husband engineered a toggle switch so I could use the turn signals without letting go of the control.
>
> "We have a *used* van with a chair lift. My husband plans to wire a second battery into the van with an isolator as in RV's. The lift will run off the "spare," the van off the regular battery. Neither wiring project is complicated. I will connect the two batteries together to jump start the van with double the power in the middle of a Montana winter!"

She planned to wear out her wheelchair considerably and get sand in her wheels on the trip. You don't need to spend a fortune on dependable transportation. The

money you saved buying the used van can pay for trips
to see the world!

Handicapped Parking

Handicapped parking can make the difference between going out and staying home. Contact the state
police for information about disabled parking permits
and license plates, so you can use those spaces. There is,
of course, one common problem: Lazy or uncaring able
bodied people use handicapped spaces too. When you
encounter someone violating the law, you can:

> 1) Call the police and give them the license
> plate number, or—
> 2) Display severe, visible disability as you
> struggle from your car next to the disabled
> space.

You can also confront the violator directly, but this
more often makes him self righteous and angry, not
penitent. The police have the authority to convince the
violator of his error. Some of you may think my second
solution rather shoddy. It *is* shoddy, but it's also *fun*!

Community Access and You

Now that you have created a safe, comfortable roll-
around home for yourself, you are ready to drive
downtown for a day of shopping, browsing, working or
whatever. But wait! Have you planned your route?
Which buildings are accessible? Where will you eat
lunch? Where are the accessible bathrooms and the
smooth curb cuts? If your downtown is not perfectly
accessible, must you stay home?

You grew up as a healthy, erect person. You still can
remember the erect person's perspective on disability

and architectural barriers. Now you are in a position to educate other people about your new needs. You are learning about what should be done to make buildings accessible, and when a curb cut should be replaced. Make yourself available, so tomorrow will be better for you and for that significant percentage of today's erect citizens, who will be wheelers tomorrow.

Note: Figures 3-3, 3-4, 3-5, 3-7, 3-10, 3-12. 3-14, and 3-18 are reproduced with permission from the American National Standards Institute.

ADDRESSES

1) *Accent on Living.* P.O. Box 700, Bloomington, Il, 61701. Published quarterly. Price: $6.00 per year.

2) *Paraplegia News.* 5201 North 19th Ave., Suite 111, Phoenix, AZ, 85015. Published monthly. Price $12.00 per year.

3) American National Standards Institute, 1430 Broadway, New York, N.Y., 10018. The ANSI Standard A117.1, 1980 costs $8.00.

Section Two

Management of MS Symptoms

Introduction

MS cannot be removed by miracles or good ideas, but the burden of disability can be eased through effective management. I have written each chapter in this section as though symptoms exist in isolation, even though I know they do not. Editor Mary Talbo emphasized the complexity of MS management after she finished reading draft copies of this section:

> "In real life every task poses many problems. When I prepare food from my wheelchair, I have no access to shelves in an upper cupboard, or food on the top shelf of the refrigerator. Carrying liquids from one end of the room to the other, opening cans, getting dishes from the cupboard; each requires more strength than I have.
>
> "Even going to the bathroom requires planning. In the chapter on bladder management, you mention that someone can't go out to play bridge because the bathroom is too far away. Those of us in wheelchairs may not even be able to get into the *house*! You deal with the mechanics of bladder management, but you don't mention that it requires planning to get to the toilet in the first place. Is the doorway wide enough? How will I transfer to the toilet? How will I get clothing out of the way and find dexterity to take down and return zippers?
>
> "Healthy people think a place is accessible if there is only one step up or down. If the bathroom is on the same floor, they think it is accessible. If it looks big enough inside, it's

accessible, even though the door is too narrow to let the chair into the room in the first place! Sometimes I stay home just because there is such a risk in going out.

"I have learned that *no* book can give all the answers. I am determined to run my own life and find ways to circumvent symptoms that interfere! When I can't find the way, even though it's hard, I ask for help. Asking allows me to retain control of my life, and keeps me fighting so this disease can't make me an invalid."

If you learn that one lesson from Mary Talbo and this book, *that you can run your own life,* we have done our job. People are more effective when they tackle disability one small chunk at a time. They combine individual management practices for easiest mobility, best access, least embarrassment, and most fun. It may be hard to discover the right combination. Our goal is to start you off in the right direction.

As Mary Talbo says, this book cannot answer all your questions. It *can* get you started on the complicated process of management. Absorb everything you can about management of individual symptoms. Find combinations of management techniques that work. Then teach the rest of us what you know, step by step, so your MSer colleagues can become better managers, and your friends and family better companions and helpers tomorrow.

Chapter 4
Management of Spasticity
John K. Wolf

Spasticity is a major problem of MS. Your spastic legs will become more comfortable once you discover a proper dose of medication, and an effective dosage schedule. Learn to use Lioresal® (baclofen) or Dantrium® (dantrolene) if you have significant spasticity.

Diagnosis of spasticity is not difficult. An ankle bounces uncontrollably on the floor or footrest. That is clonus. A leg jerks suddenly, or thighs jerk the knees toward each other when they should be separated. Those are spastic spasms. Leg muscles feel tight and stiff as you walk, and rapidly become fatigued and painful. Movements of fingers and limbs are slowed. Grip is imperfect and standing balance suffers. Spasticity interferes with *all* movements. Spasticity eventually produces loss of power and sometimes total paralysis. Spasticity is a major cause of exhaustion among MSers.

Tightness

Exhaustion

Clonus

Spontaneous spasms

Pain

Slowed reaction time

Imbalance

Loss of power

Paralysis

In the absence of spasticity, these symptoms often occur individually. When the pyramidal tract (See Fig. 17-2, page 307) is damaged anywhere in its path from the brain to the spinal cord, they occur together. An examiner discovers *hyper*active deep tendon reflexes and often a Babinski sign. (See page 314.) Lioresal or Dantrium can effectively stop clonus and spasms, loosen the tightness, relieve pain, improve balance, make walking easier and significantly lessen fatigue. No medication brings back lost power, but muscle strengthening exercises are easier and more effective with help from antispastic medication.

LIORESAL® (Baclofen)

Chemistry and Mechanism of Action

Baclofen was first formulated by chemists at CIBA - GEIGY, Ltd., who were looking for a compound to diminish muscle tightness. Gamma Amino Butyric Acid (GABA) performs some of this function in the spinal cord, but GABA cannot be used as a medication because, taken by mouth, or even intravenously, GABA does not enter the central nervous system. CIBA - GEIGY chemists formulated a number of compounds similar to GABA. Of these only baclofen resulted in useful reduction of spasticity (Fig. 4-1). Once it was found to be effective, baclofen was given the Trade Name, Lioresal®.

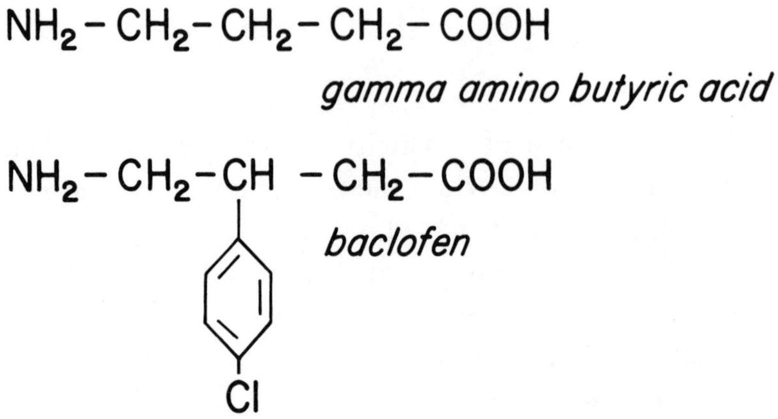

$$NH_2 - CH_2 - CH_2 - CH_2 - COOH$$

gamma amino butyric acid

$$NH_2 - CH_2 - CH - CH_2 - COOH$$

baclofen

Cl

Fig. 4-1. Chemical structure of GABA (top) and Lioresal® (bottom). No knowledge of organic chemistry is needed to recognize the similarity of these two chemicals.

An oral dose of Lioresal is rapidly absorbed from the intestinal tract and moves rapidly to the brain and spinal cord. Apart from its action in reducing spasticity, it is almost inert. It does not participate in the chemical reactions of the body and is rapidly excreted in the urine and feces. This inactivity is beneficial because Lioresal has few cross reactions with other medications. Indeed, the major disadvantage of Lioresal results from its speedy transit through the body. Lioresal is absorbed and excreted so fast that its biological half-life is only two to four hours.

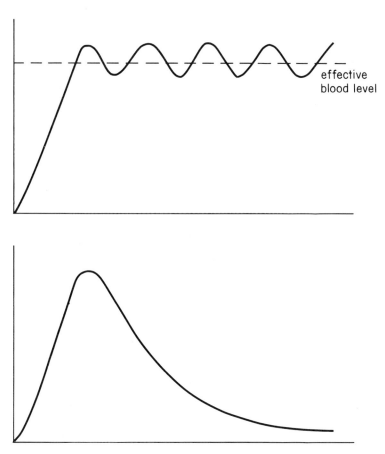

effective
blood level

Fig. 4-2. Effect of dosage frequency on blood levels. Frequent small doses (top) maintain a steady blood level, even though the biological half-life is short. Infrequent large doses provide inconsistent control of spasticity.

Biological Half-Life

The biological half-life of medications determines dosage schedules. Imagine a medication that is rapidly absorbed but remains active for many days. Such a medication has a long biological half-life. Were there no initial side effects, one could take a loading dose to build up an effective concentration in the body, and then a daily maintenance dose to maintain a proper level. Most antidepressants, for example, have long biological half-lives. Their concentration in the body increases for about two weeks after a person begins to take a daily dose. Eventually the amount of medicine destroyed or excreted in a day equals the daily dose, and the concentration in the body remains stable.

Now imagine a medication like Lioresal, which is absorbed and excreted rapidly. The effect of a single dose lasts only minutes or hours. Lioresal has a *short* biological half-life. If such a medication is to have continuous effectiveness it must be taken several times in 24 hours.

Biological half-life and effective blood and tissue levels are two major determinants of a medication's effectiveness. If the total daily dose is too small, its concentration in the blood will not rise high enough to be effective. If the biological half-life is short, a more frequent dosage schedule is required to maintain constant levels in blood and tissues (Fig. 4-2).

The usual biological half-life of Lioresal is two to four hours. In some people the biological half-life may be as long as five or even six hours, in others as short as an hour. Thus, *some MSers can take Lioresal as infrequently as three times in 24 hours while some others must take a dose 12 times a day on a regular two-hour schedule in order to maintain constant control of spastic symptoms.*

Effect of Lioresal on Spasticity

Lioresal is especially useful for MSers because it relieves spasticity caused by spinal cord lesions. Much MS spasticity comes from plaques in that part of the nervous system. A proper dose and dosage schedule of Lioresal will remove unwanted muscle spasms, lessen fatigue and improve gait. But effective as it is, Lioresal is still an imperfect answer to MS gait disturbance. It does not improve muscle power and has no effect on the imbalance and incoordination caused by cerebellar or sensory malfunction.

Lioresal *is* effective in relieving that part of the gait disturbance caused by leg spasticity. Walking depends on gross movements of large muscles. Tightness of these muscles is relieved by Lioresal. Lioresal is less effective in improving function of hands and arms. Accurate fine finger movements depend on precision of neuronal function, which is unchanged by Lioresal.

The best result from Lioresal occurs in the severely disabled MSer who is confined to bed or wheelchair by spastic paralysis. In this instance Lioresal is truly a minor miracle. The best dose produces floppy, limp legs that transfer more easily from bed to chair and toilet. This dose relieves painful spasms. It allows the legs to relax so groin and bottom may be washed. Care of bowel and bladder function is made easier. Use of Lioresal in this situation will not make you walk again, but it will make you much more comfortable.

Many people now have medical insurance that pays for prescriptions. Lioresal is very expensive if you must pay for each tablet. Lioresal is ineffective unless there is significant spastic muscle tightness. So don't ask for a Lioresal prescription unless your life is significantly disturbed by symptoms of spasticity. Ask your neurologist whether your neurological examination supports your conclusion. If not, read another part of this book that has more value to you now. Come back to this chapter when you have more trouble.

Finding Your Best Dose

Each person must establish the proper dose and dosage schedule through use. The "best dose" of

Lioresal produces the best improvement in walking, balance, spasms and fatigue. Lioresal comes in 10 mg. and 20 mg. scored tablets. Begin by taking 5 mg. every six hours and increase the dose by 5 mg. per dose every three days until you approach your best dose.

As Lioresal begins to work, spontaneous spasms stop. With each dosage increase, muscles become looser. Finally, when you have gone *beyond* your best dose, loose muscles feel weak and heavy. This side effect begins 30–60 minutes after the most recent dose. But it lasts only an hour or two because of the brief biological half-life. This is the signal that you have passed your best dosage level. Now, search for your *best* dose. It will usually be smaller by five to 15 mg. per dose.

Always begin at five mg. every six hours. Occasional MSers reach their best dose at a level of 10–20 mg. per 24 hours, but most MSers find their best dose in the range of 120–160 mg. per day. This is almost double the 80 mg. per day recommended by the Food and Drug Administration. That regulation is the result of testing protocols that were arbitrarily limited to 80 mg. per day. No one has done a precise evaluation of the side effects of larger doses. MSers regularly exceed that dose without severe side effects and regularly receive inadequate relief from spasticity at lower dosage levels.

Avoid the common errors of Lioresal use. Remember the brief biological half-life and use Lioresal at least four times in 24 hours. Remember that you are looking for your *best* dose, not simply for improvement. Increase your dose until you know that you have gone beyond *best* into mild side effects of *too much*. Then reduce it to your best dose, confident that you have really gotten the most from the medication.

Once you have reached your best dose in this manner, adjust the dose to fit daily variations in symptoms. Adjust the dosage schedule to fit your life. Check your dose periodically, to be certain it still is the best dose for you.

Change the Dose to Fit Your Symptoms

Do you have more spasms in the afternoon than the morning? Increase the noon dose to fit your afternoon needs.

Are you going on a trip in the wheelchair today, which will bounce you around and cause more spasms? To prevent that complication, take extra Lioresal before you leave. Are there whole days when you are more spastic? Alter the dose each day to fit your needs.

Change Dosage Schedules to Fit your life

You aren't awake at 6:00 A.M., 12:00 noon, 6:00 P.M. and midnight? Then take a larger dose when you go to bed for a long sleep. Do you wake in the middle of the night with increasing spasticity, because the time is too long between bedtime and morning? Use the state of your spasticity to tell what time it is, as other MSers do, and take an extra dose in the middle of the night to tide you over till morning. Either plan allows you to have more Lioresal in your blood when you wake up, in order to avoid early morning spasticity.

Does each dose begin to wear off in four hours rather than six? In two hours? Then change the dosage schedule to keep the effect of Lioresal constant during the entire 24 hours. Many MSers take Lioresal every four hours, and a few take Lioresal every two hours throughout the day and night.

Check Your Dose Periodically, to be Sure it's Still Right

The best dose when you first start Lioresal, may not be your best dose forever. As your spasticity changes, your need for Lioresal will also change. Check periodically, to see whether yours is still the best dose. Decrease it for several days to see if you feel better. Then increase it for a few days to see if you develop weak, heavy arms and legs. Readjust your dose to fit your comfort. If you fail to check, you will never know that your body requirements have changed!

Side Effects of Lioresal

Drowsiness, the most common side effect of Lioresal, results when Lioresal impairs nervous system function above the spinal cord. Excitement and even seizures have been reported but are uncommon. One of my own patients developed psychological depression and could not use Lioresal at all. Sometimes Lioresal upsets the stomach. Side effects are less bothersome if the dose is increased gradually. Lioresal will not be useful if you are incapacitated by side effects, so take your time. If you become sleepy, wait at that dosage level to see if it will pass. Increase the dose again only if side effects disappear. You will be better satisfied with the end result.

Lioresal is largely ineffective in the treatment of a spastic bladder. However, Lioresal may aggravate borderline dysfunction in a partially flaccid bladder and cause urinary retention.

It is uncomfortable and occasionally dangerous to stop Lioresal suddenly once the dose has been raised to effective levels. The resulting sudden return of spasticity may be very painful. More serious side effects such as hallucinations have been reported. Should you decide to stop Lioresal, plan to taper the dose toward zero over a week or ten day period.

The Emergency Supply

To prevent sudden withdrawl from Lioresal or from any other useful medication, hide a two week emergency supply of all your medications in the back of the medicine cabinet separate from the daily supply. Then if your pharmacist has run out and must order your medications, or if you carelessly run out of pills on Saturday night, simply bring out the emergency supply and use it until you refill your prescriptions.

Once you have refilled the prescription, *replace the tablets you used* from the emergency supply so they will be there when you need them again. Rotate your emergency supply with the active supply so your emergency tablets do not become outdated on the shelf.

Warnings

The only direct contraindication to the use of Lioresal is an established allergy to it.

MSers with kidney disease may need a smaller daily dose and perhaps less frequent dosage schedules. Remember, Lioresal is excreted primarily through the kidneys. Begin with a smaller dose if you have kidney failure, perhaps 5 mg. every 12 hours. Increase the dose less rapidly, perhaps every week. Remember that if excretion is slowed, biological half-life is increased, so toxic side effects of flaccid looseness also last longer than usual.

There is no accurate information about the effects of Lioresal on the developing fetus. Pregnant women should avoid Lioresal, and other medications if possible, during at least the first four months of pregnancy.

DANTRIUM® (Dantrolene)

Some MSers cannot tolerate Lioresal. Perhaps the effect of even modest reduction of spasticity worsens the gait disturbance, so antispastic medications are of no value. Perhaps Lioresal causes such overwhelming sleepiness, upset stomach or other side effect that it cannot be tolerated, even though reduction of spasticity *could* be valuable. The MSer who cannot take Lioresal but has significant spasticity should consider Dantrium®.

Mechanism of Action

Dantrium works in the depths of the muscle fiber, at the farthest end of the muscle contraction mechanism. Once the electrochemical message reaches the muscle membrane it is transmitted into the the muscle cell by membranous tubules that release calcium ions through special pores in their walls. These calcium ions begin the process of muscle contraction at the level of the contractile protein molecules within the muscle cell. Dantrium reduces release of calcium ions through the pores and thus reduces muscle tightness.

Warning and Side Effects

Dantrium is potentially toxic. It is recommended only for significant spasticity that does not respond to Lioresal. Serious side effects are uncommon but liver damage caused by Dantrium may be fatal. Before you consider using Dantrium have blood studies to test liver function. Avoid Dantrium completely if there is evidence of active liver disease of any kind, or cirrhosis from any cause. Once treatment with Dantrium is begun, have liver function monitored every week or two while the dose. is being increased, and less frequently once the best dose is established.

Liver toxicity occurs more frequently among patients who use more than 800 mg. per day, more frequently in women and more frequently in those over 35 years of age. Although severe liver damage is uncommon, it occurs often enough that Dantrium cannot be recommended for treatment of trivial symptoms. Discontinue Dantrium if it is ineffective or only marginally effective at the best dose.

There is no accurate information about the effects of Dantrium on the developing fetus. Pregnant women should avoid Dantrium and other medications if possible, during at least the first four months of pregnancy.

Every treatment has undesirable side effects that must be balanced against potential benefits. It is usually worthwhile to cross the street despite the small chance of being run down by a truck. MSers with severe spasticity who have tried Lioresal and could not use it, and whose blood studies disclose no evidence of liver disease, might derive great benefit from the use of Dantrium. If Dantrium is effective in reducing spasticity, one might conclude that the benefit is worth the small risk of even fatal side effects. Fortunately, most readers have no need to make this choice because Lioresal is so consistently effective.

Use of Dantrium in Multiple Sclerosis

Dantrium comes in 25 mg., 50 mg. and 100 mg. capsules, and, for MSers who cannot easily swallow capsules, in Dantrium suspension, 25 mg. per teaspoonful. Use of any suspension is hazardous, because suspended medication particles tend to settle to the bottom of the bottle. Unless the bottle is shaken vigorously every time it is used, the result is undermedication at the beginning of the bottle and overdose at the end. *Always shake the bottle well.*

The biological half-life of Dantrium is eight to 10 hours, so the dosage schedule may be set at twice or three times in 24 hours. The effective dose varies widely. Some MSers find their best dose at less than 100 mg. per day. Others require more than 1000 mg. per day. Many MSers find that Dantrium is ineffective at any dose, so they stop it completely.

The principle is the same as with Lioresal. Begin at a small dose, 25 mg. twice a day. Remember the longer biological half-life which requires longer to stabilize the blood level. Increase the dose at weekly intervals by 25–50 mg. per day. Increase the dose as you would with Lioresal, to the point of flaccid looseness. (See pages 89–90.) Once you have reached this dosage level, reduce subsequent doses stepwise to discover the dose that produces the least fatigue, the fewest muscle spasms and the best overall function.

OTHER TREATMENTS FOR SPASTICITY

Valium® (diazepam) has been used for treatment of spasticity but it is largely ineffective. Chronic use may be habit forming and may lead to serious abuse. Avoid Valium except for an occasional tablet for some exceptional reason, usually "nervousness." Then use it sparingly.

One exception to this advice has come to my attention. A young man made paraplegic by a motorcycle accident had spastic spasms so severe that they actually threw him from his wheelchair. On a dose of Lioresal,

25 mg. every three hours around the clock (200 mg. per day), his spasms abated significantly. When we then added Valium 5 mg. four times a day to the regimen, his legs became limp. This was a completely satisfactory regimen for him. His was an unusually severe degree of spasticity. It is probably unduplicated among MSers, but for those with severe spasticity, the combination should be considered.

Much more aggressive treatments for spasticity have been used, but these should be considered only for severe spastic paralysis that has not responded to medications. Consult your neurologist or neurosurgeon about such procedures and plan to avoid them unless yours is an exceptional case.

DO NOT "GO IT ALONE." KEEP IN TOUCH.

Lioresal, Dantrium and most other medications discussed in this volume are prescription drugs designed for specific use. I have attempted to outline effective methods for discovering proper doses and dosage schedules, but written words cannot substitute for conversations. Use your doctor as you begin to investigate new medications. Even if these particular ones are unfamiliar to your physician, their use is similar to other medications. The doctor can give you more individual advice on their use than you can get from these pages alone.

Chapter 5
Bladder Management
By John K. Wolf

Bladder symptoms are manageable. You need not be incontinent. Urgency and frequency can be reduced. Bladder infection can usually be prevented. If you want to go to church or to synagogue, to a friend's house for bridge, if you want to travel, do it. Carry your bladder management practices with you. You must spend extra time each day thinking about bladder function, but the time will be well spent because it will lead to more personal freedom.

Decide now that you will never tolerate urinary incontinence. Learn to control or circumvent bladder and bowel dysfunction. Start now so you will have time to master each new problem one step at a time before the next one arrives. Never let things slide. If you learn management early and keep learning new techniques as they become valuable, you will never suddenly require a complex new regimen that cannot easily be mastered.

This chapter is especially important for junior MSers who may have no experience with bladder malfunction. If you are a junior MSer, read this chapter for information, not for practice. Learn that there are solutions to problems of bladder dysfunction, and that *prompt atten-*

tion to first symptoms can prevent long term complications.

Senior MSers may already know most of these management techniques. If you have long experience, learn whatever new ideas this chapter has to offer, and continue those practices that allow you to maintain your composure and mobility.

Notice

A discussion of the anatomy of bladder function is available on pages 317–322. I encourage you to read it if you wish to broaden your understanding of bladder symptoms.

RESIDUAL URINE VOLUME DETERMINES MANAGEMENT PRACTICES

Normal bladders empty completely. MS bladders often do not. The *residual urine volume* is the amount of urine left in the bladder after voiding. This is the major determinant of bladder management.

Large Residual Volume Encourages Infection

Imagine the plight of bacteria that attempt to invade a normal bladder. After they climb the urethra to reach the bladder, they face frequent tidal flows of urine, from completely full, to completely empty. New bacteria that collect between voidings are washed out every time the normal bladder empties. Bladder infection is rare among healthy people because bacteria cannot gain a foothold.

Now imagine the delight of bacteria, if they *could* delight, upon their arrival in a bladder with a large residual urine volume and the small volume variations that characterize purely flaccid and MS bladders. After working their way up the urethra, they fall into a warm, nutritious lake with a trickle tube at the outflow. A few of them are washed out with each voiding, but the others multiply happily in the residual urine volume. As bacteria multiply in the urine, they begin to invade the bladder wall, causing cystitis. Inflammation of the bladder wall results in pain, urgency and frequency. The bacteria cause cloudy, smelly urine.

How Big is Big?

How large a residual is dangerous? There is no firm answer. Most people with a residual urine volume less than 100 cc. (3–4 ounces) have no trouble. Larger residual urine volumes are riskier. Bladder infection is more of a problem for women than men. The female urethra is shorter and runs along the front wall of the vagina where repeated pressure during sexual intercourse forces bacteria into the bladder. Women without sexual partners have fewer infections. But I don't recommend this option as a first line of defense against infection!

Repeated Infection Causes Scarring

White blood cells enter the bladder wall to combat the bacterial infection. Afterward, products of inflammation remain in the bladder wall as scars that grow with each subsequent infection. Scar tissue reduces the normal stretching and contracting of the bladder wall. Scars are permanent. They are also *preventable* through careful management. But they cannot easily be *treated*.

Neglected bladders that become scarred and distended occasionally develop abnormal outpouchings in the wall. These are called diverticulae. A diverticulum does not contract. It becomes a permanent part of the residual urine volume. It forms a perfect site for bacteria and sediment to collect. (Fig. 5-1). These complications of cystitis are serious, but preventable, by early recognition and treatment of increased residual urine volume, and of bladder infections.

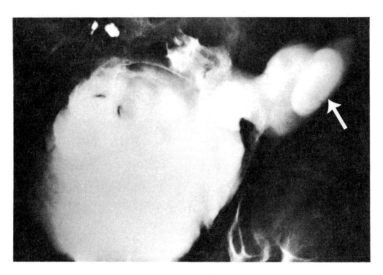

Fig. 5-1. Bladder diverticulae. These pockets (arrow) never empty. They result from neglect. They can be prevented by careful management.

DIAGNOSIS AND TREATMENT OF URINARY TRACT INFECTION

Proper management helps to prevent infection, but even the best management techniques may fail. Infection remains the most common serious complication of bladder dysfunction, especially among junior MSers who deny that it can happen to them. Junior MSers remain primarily concerned about the problems of frequency and urgency, not about constant and careful management. Usually this attitude has no serious consequences. The first bladder infection does little damage if it is diagnosed, treated and followed promptly by effective management practices.

Diagnosis of Bladder Infection

The usual symptoms of bladder infection are urgency, frequency and pain on urination. There is a dull ache in the lower abdomen. Women complain of vaginal tenderness. Because of sensory loss many MSers cannot depend on these symptoms as warning signals. Instead, MSers must rely on nose, eyes and thermometer for diagnosis. Bacteria in the urine produce bad smelling by-products. Bacteria and white cells in the urine make it cloudy. Finally, if those symptoms are ignored, fever and prostration follow. These signify a serious, life-threatening bladder infection. When your urine begins to smell and looks cloudy, assume that you have an infection. Call your doctor immediately.

A urine sample for culture is taken during the middle of urination. Most of the organisms living in the urethra are washed out with the first ounce or so. Discard that first portion. Then collect two to four tablespoonsful of urine in a clean jar. Take the sample immediately to the doctor's office or the laboratory for urinalysis and culture.

Urinalysis

Once it arrives in the laboratory, the sample is poured into a test tube. It is spun down in a centrifuge to concentrate bacteria and white cells as sediment in the bottom of the tube. The intensity of the body's reaction to infection is estimated by a count of the white blood cells in the sediment. Normally nothing but an occasional white cell and a few strings of mucus are visible under the microscope. In slow-moving infections, bacteria may be visible, but few white cells. If the infection is "red hot" and the body defenses are up, many white cells have entered the urine and can be seen under the microscope, combatting infection as best they can.

Urine Culture and Sensitivity

Part of the urine specimen goes directly to the bacteriology laboratory, where bacteria are grown on culture plates. Each kind of culture medium encourages the growth of certain kinds of bacteria and discourages others. These and certain other growth characteristics allow precise identification of the organism. Most bacteria grow fast enough to form visible colonies on the culture medium in 24 hours, and different kinds of bacteria form colonies of different color and size. Samples from selected colonies can then be plated out once more in the presence of several antibiotics to determine which will be most effective.

If your symptoms suggest infection, your doctor may start treatment as soon as you deliver the sample. The urinalysis provides information about the organism and gives limited guidance in the choice of antibiotic. After one day the urine culture identifies the organism. By the second or third day your response to treatment, and the results of antibiotic sensitivity tests, confirm the choice of antibiotic.

Even appropriate antibiotic therapy fails to sterilize the urine in enlarged, flaccid bladders. If a bladder infection does not subside promptly, even though treated with antibiotics chosen to combat the causative organism, the reason is probably *high residual urine volume*. If the infection clears up rapidly but symptoms return in a week or two, the cause is high residual urine volume *plus* poor management. For proper management at this point, increase fluid intake, acidify the urine, do the best Credé you can, and take another course of the antibiotic. This may be adequate, but if the infection returns anyway, you will probably need at least several weeks of self-cath to bring the bladder back to its normal size and to start your planned management program. Let's examine simple techniques first, before discussing self-cath.

EASY BLADDER MANAGEMENT TECHNIQUES

The goals of bladder management are the same for everyone: That the bladder empty *completely* on command, that it empty *only* on command and that complications of urinary tract dysfunction be avoided.

Learn basic bladder management as soon as any symptom of bladder dysfunction appears. Strive constantly for perfection. Plan to learn new techniques as soon as they become useful. You need learn only a few techniques, but each has its place in the scheme of bladder management. The simple ones include maintenance of high daily urine volume, acidification of the urine, Credé and double voidings.

Maintenance of High Daily Urine Volume

Urinary frequency and incontinence are a terrible burden, but water restriction is a poor solution to the problem. Low daily urine volume allows bacteria to multiply in a stagnant bladder. Mucus and debris are not washed out. Bladder stones form more easily in concentrated urine. Feces in the colon become dry and hard. Avoid fluid restriction as a cure for urinary frequency.

Fluid restriction in the evening after supper is quite acceptable if it leads to a more peaceful night and is counterbalanced by large fluid intake during waking

104

hours. Occasional fluid restriction during the day is also acceptable, but don't overdo it.

Are you traveling to Chicago by plane? Do you plan a trip on the freeway today? Drink less for breakfast and dehydrate yourself for the trip. But make up for the loss when you arrive. Your goal is to have more normal bladder function with adequate daily fluid intake, without the complications of infection and sediments. Plan to drink enough to maintain an average urine volume of *at least* two quarts per day.

Maintenance of Acid Urine

Acidify the urine to prevent bladder infection. Most bladder bacteria thrive in alkaline urine, but are inhibited by acid. Vitamin C acidifies the urine if taken in a large enough dose. It is available without prescription in 500 mg. tablets at any pharmacy. Special urinary acidifying medications are available with prescription.

Test your urine for acidity. If you are lucky, your pharmacist may have pH paper. Combistix® are more expensive. They cost about $.25 per Combistick, but each one is wide enough to be cut in half lengthwise with a razor or scissors. Acid urine has a pH below 7.0. The pH of alkaline urine is above that number. Establish your proper dose of vitamin C by aiming for a urinary pH below 6.5. Most people need four to eight grams per day (eight to sixteen 500 mg. tablets) in divided doses. Take a gram of vitamin C (two 500 mg. tablets) morning, noon and evening for several days to start. Three or four days later, check the pH of your urine and change the dose accordingly.

Cranberry juice contains large quantities of vitamin C, but it is expensive. If you use too much it can cause diarrhea. Fred Krauss (See Dedication, page v.) found the perfect combination: liberal quantities of cranberry juice, mixed with restrained quantities of vodka. It kept his urine acid and his disposition sweet!

If vitamin C acidification fails to prevent infection, or if you cannot use it for some other reason, Uroqid-Acid®, available by prescription, combines urinary acidification with methenamine. Methenamine releases formaldehyde in an acid urine, further suppressing bacterial growth. K-Phos M.F.® tablets provide urinary acidification without methenamine. If you use such preparations, maintain your urine pH below 6.5 for best effect. Consult your doctor about contraindications to the use of these medications.

Credé Maneuver

Successful Credé increases the tidal variation between completely full, and as empty as possible. Credé does not empty the MS bladder. It merely improves emptying by forcing excess urine from an enlarged, flaccid bladder. Use of Credé also helps to prevent further bladder enlargement by allowing the bladder wall to contract between voidings. If you wonder whether your bladder is enlarged, have a professional examine your abdomen. If the bladder is palpable, Credé may help.

Many MSers discover Credé without instruction. Sit on the toilet or commode and relax your abdominal wall. Press inward and downward. Can you feel the mass of an enlarged bladder? If bladder sensation is intact, you also feel urgency or a desire to void as you press down harder. Begin to urinate and push forcibly inward and downward, rolling your fist into the abdominal wall against the bladder. Did you hear a gush of urine? Follow it right down as far as you can into the pelvis, forcing out as much urine as possible.

People with enlarged bladders who have trouble learning Credé often have not pressed hard enough on the top of the bladder, or have failed to pursue the emptying bladder down into the pelvic cavity. In some cases, Credé fails because the bladder neck goes into involuntary spasm during the maneuver. If you press *hard* and remain unsuccessful, this may be your trouble. In this case, Credé is not for you just now. Try Dibenzyline®. (See page 121.) It may give you relief. Should your bladder function change in the future, Credé still might become an effective management technique, so don't discard it permanently.

If you are obese or weak-handed, Credé may be ineffective because you simply cannot push hard enough on the dome of the bladder. Another technique may work better. Try leaning forward on the toilet, grasping your two hands under your thighs. Take a deep breath and push. Pull down with your arms and listen for the effect down below. Be careful not to lose your balance in this position. Either technique for Credé may be useful for quite another reason. A woman from Watertown, N.Y., reports that Credé improves emptying of her bowels. She presses her filled bladder against the colon as she Credés and empties bladder and bowels together.

Double Voidings can Improve Emptying

Double voiding gives your bladder a chance to empty more completely than it otherwise would. Urinate. Use whatever kind of Credé works for you. Then get up and do something else for a few minutes. This wait allows a tired bladder to contract down on its residual urine volume and to get ready for another try. One woman said she stands up and jumps up and down several times before sitting down to try once more. Her jumping has the same effect as massaging the bladder wall. It alerts the sacral spinal cord so it can do its job more effectively.

ROADMAP THROUGH FANCIER TECHNIQUES OF BLADDER MANAGEMENT

Usually, the presence of bladder flaccidity alone is not an adequate reason to learn self-cath. If your bladder is enlarged, but you are living with it successfully, learn what's necessary to keep it from becoming larger. Learn Credé. Consider Dibenzyline® (See page 121.) if you have severe hesitancy. Use the other easy management techniques listed above, but do not bother with self-cath yet.

If you have had no bladder infection, but you have significant spasticity in the legs and urinary urgency and frequency, you may also have a spastic component to bladder function. If so, learn to use Ditropan® . Go to page 117 for discussion of management practices for bladder spasticity.

If, in addition to bladder spasms and severe urgency, you must wait many minutes before you can actually urinate, you may have detrusor-sphincter dyssynergia. This topic is discussed on page 121.

In any case, read this chapter and then discuss your situation with your physician before you begin any treatment. If you want more information about the anatomy of bladder control, read pages 317–322 in

Chapter 17. Get information from all sources, and then learn effective management practices.

MANAGEMENT OF BLADDER FLACCIDITY

A flaccid bladder often signals its presence. The *first difference* MSers detect is *abdominal fullness*. I ask whether the MSer can express more urine by pressing down on the lower abdomen. (See Credé maneuver, page 106.) MSers with flaccid bladders often reply that they have already found that this works. Cheryl Krauzer from Derry, New Hampshire, wrote that she thought she had invented this maneuver until she read the first edition of *Mastering Multiple Sclerosis*. Many other MSers must have duplicated her experience. Unfortunately, not all MSers with enlarged bladders can Credé successfully: the bladder neck goes into spasm as they try, or they have too much hand weakness or are obese. If you believe your bladder is enlarged, but Credé has been ineffective, ask your doctor for an examination to discover if you are right.

The *second difference* is *bladder infection*, which is often the first definite sign of a flaccid bladder. Spastic bladders are constantly busy emptying themselves and rarely become infected. Flaccid bladders are a reservoir with a perfect culture medium, ready and waiting for bacteria to arrive. If you have already had bladder infection and Credé effectively expresses more urine, or if you can feel the enlarged bladder looming up above the pelvis, you have bladder flaccidity. Begin management with Credé and other simple management practices discussed above. But if bladder infection returns anyway, learn self-cath. Then you can monitor and control your own residual urine volume, and avoid many complications.

Self-Catheterization

Some MSers live successful uninfected lives despite large residual urine volumes. They manage incontinence with adult diapers or by cutting disposable diapers in half and using them as safety pads. Some use sanitary napkins successfully. Usually, however, diapers and sanitary napkins are a poor solution because of constant wetness and odor. When skin remains wet, bedsores are more likely to develop over pressure areas. If simple things don't work, like diapers or condom drainage, maybe self-cath will.

I usually do not recommend self-cath until after the first bladder infection, because some MSers have no complications despite very large residuals. It is important to prevent the return of old complications, but there is no need to ask for *new* ones.

Your doctor can help you decide. In addition to providing an assessment of bladder function, your doctor can arrange for a professional at the office, in the hospital or in your own home, to teach you self-cath. With professional help, you will have an easier start, and will learn more quickly and easily.

By mastering self-cath and keeping a record of the residual urine volumes, you regain control of your own bladder function. If you check your own residual urine volume regularly, you can *decide* how large you will allow it to become. Did infection arrive at a residual of 150 cc? Then keep your residuals below 100 cc. If the residual climbs above your chosen limit, and yours is not a badly scarred or damaged bladder, repeated self-cath at four to six hour intervals will again bring it down. When self-cath is done regularly for a few days to two weeks after the first urinary tract infection, residuals almost always return to normal. Then the catheter can be put away for once-a-week use, to monitor the residual and keep it at a proper volume.

Even if the residuals are not reduced after doing self-cath every four to six hours, the procedure empties the bladder completely each time, and repeatedly prevents the return of infection and its complications. Self-cath allows you to empty your bladder and go out on the town with confidence, knowing that the catheter is safely tucked into a pocket or purse, where it is ready for use at the slightest feeling of need, or at a timed interval. You can use public toilets as you did before you got MS. With self-cath, you have once more improved your well-being.

There is no need to boil your hands before doing self-cath. Learn it as a *clean* procedure, not a *sterile* one. Run water through the catheter after each use and wash it occasionally with soap. Once it has dried, keep it in a pouch or any clean container where it will be handy. Do not make your bladder management so difficult that it loses its value.

Some people cannot perform self-cath. Severe tremor, excessive obesity, paralysis or sensory loss in the hands prevent successful self-cath. If you have incontinence from a flaccid bladder but cannot self-cath, condom drainage works well for some men. Indwelling catheters or diapers work well for other men and for women.

Self-Cath for Men

Self-cath is easy for men. The penis is readily available. Use a 16 French* plain catheter. Lubricate the tip

---

* Catheters are graded according to size by French units. One French unit is one-third millimeter, so a 15 Fr. catheter has a five mm. diameter, a 24 Fr. catheter, eight mm.

of the catheter with *water soluble* lubricating jelly available at any pharmacy. Do *not* use petroleum jelly, which
is insoluble. Hold the penis perpendicular to the body
and insert the tip of the catheter into the urethral
opening. Pass the catheter forward into the bladder and
voilà, a gusher! Resistance occurs as the tip passes
through the prostate gland (Fig. 5-2). When you feel this
resistance, simply keep pushing gently until the tip slips
through the prostatic urethra and falls into the bladder.
Self cath is not painful, but as the catheter passes
through the prostate, you may feel its passage as a
sudden almost sexual "rush."

There is one anatomical problem you should know
about, just in case. Occasionally, small glands in the
prostate enlarge to form a false passage for the catheter.
These glands trap the catheter in the substance of the
gland by diverting it from the main passage, which is
the prostatic urethra. Once this happens, no amount of
pushing can pass the catheter into the bladder. Further
manipulation will only cause swelling, pain and infection instead of relief. The immediate consequence is
urinary retention.

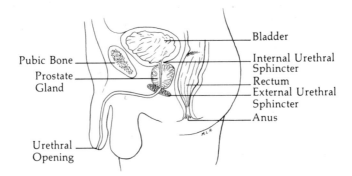

**Fig. 5-2. Male anatomy. The urethral orifice is
easily accessible. Catheter must pass through the
prostatic urethra to reach the bladder.**

This seldom happens to young men who self-cath regularly. However, if it does occur and you cannot insert the catheter, go *immediately* to the nearest emergency room for catheterization. Otherwise, the real emergency of complete urinary retention and an increasingly distended bladder will develop while you wait. Emergency room personnel will insert an indwelling catheter and suggest that you leave it in place for several days until all swelling and irritation subside.

A coudé catheter with a specially curved tip is used in this situation. The tip may be directed away from the false passage along the prostatic urethra and into the bladder. From that time on, continue to use the coudé catheter to avoid repetition of the incident.

Self-Cath for Women

Self-cath is harder for women. Most women have not seen their own urethral orifice. Many have only a vague idea where it is. An easy way to learn self-cath is to lie propped up in bed, knees supported by pillows, with a small mirror between the legs. The round cosmetic mirrors with little legs on them work perfectly. If this technique is uncomfortable, learn self cath sitting on the edge of the bed with the mirror on the floor, or on a stool between your legs. Don't forget the pan to catch your success!

Begin by examining your own anatomy. Shine a good light toward your vaginal area, and spread the labia to examine the vaginal orifice in the mirror (Fig. 5-3). Note the clitoris at the top of the vulva, *above* the pubic bone. When you press on the clitoris, you are pressing *down* on the pubic bone.

Then find the urethral orifice immediately below and tucked up behind the pubic bone. It is a small round hole about an eighth of an inch (3 mm.) in diameter. If you press on the urethral orifice, you must press *up* to reach the pubic bone. Below the urethral orifice is the vagina.

Feel with one finger along the under surface of the pubic bone. This route takes you along the front wall of the vagina and follows the course of the urethra. You cannot feel the urethra itself, since it is buried in the vaginal wall, but if you feel deeply enough into the vagina, your upward pressing finger will pass behind the pubic bone. At this point, your finger tip has reached the region of the bladder itself. That is your target. Now you are ready to do the hard part.

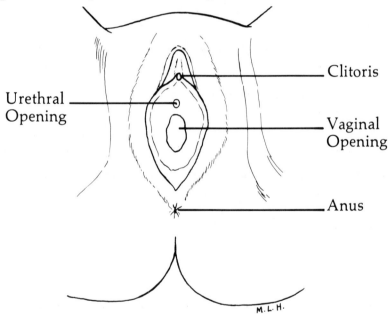

Fig. 5-3. Female anatomy. Pubic bone is not shown in the figure. Clitoris is *above* the pubic bone, urethral orifice is *below* it.

When you begin, use the same red rubber catheter men use. It is large, long and easy to hold in nervous fingers. Later your skill will improve, so you can graduate to fancier technology. I don't know how women find a way to hold the labia open with one hand, the catheter with the other, keep the light aimed right, look in the mirror without knocking it down, and still put the catheter tip into the urethra, but they do.

Lubricate the tip of the catheter with *water soluble* lubricating jelly available at any pharmacy. Do *not* use petroleum jelly, which is insoluble. Find the opening to the urethra and insert the tip. Once the tip of the catheter is in the urethra, you can relax. No more problems. No prostate to get in the way. No complications. Simply push the catheter into the bladder and let it drain.

Learn how to self-cath in bed with a mirror. Then begin to do it "blind." Then learn to do self-cath while you sit on the toilet. If you think this would be too difficult, remember that many other women have learned to do it. It is similar to inserting a tampon. The target is smaller, but the job is the same.

The shape and short length of the female urethra lend themselves to the use of pre-shaped metal sounds or plastic female catheters. These are much handier than the long red rubber catheters and fit neatly into purse or pocket. My women cath-ers prefer the plastic catheters. They cost about $2.00 and last several years.

Determine Your Residual Urine Volume with Self-Cath

The residual urine volume is the amount of urine left in the bladder after voiding. Now that you know how to self-cath, you can easily determine your own residual urine volume. Empty your bladder as completely as possible, using Credé if that works for you. Then self-cath and collect that urine in a measuring cup. Record the volume and the date so you always have the information available when you need it. Record also the symptoms you have on that date. Did you measure your residual volume because you had an infection? If so, that residual is too big! Resolve to keep your residual volume smaller than that number, and to check it regularly to be sure your bladder management plan is effective.

External Drainage

External drainage emphasizes the advantages of male anatomy. It is right there and ready to accept things that need to be attached to it. Tubing from a leg bag or night bag can be attached directly to the blind end of a condom with a rubber band. Then a hole poked in the condom over the tip of the tubing allows the urine to drain into the bag when the condom is placed over the penis. If it tends to slip off, it can be attached with Davol® rubber cement, or with a Velcro® band. If you use Velcro, be careful not to fasten it too tight. The devastating result might annihilate the advantages of male anatomy, preventing further use of this kind of drainage!

More expensive disposable condom drainage sets may be purchased at pharmacies or Physicians and Hospital Supply stores. Several companies make reusable external drainage sets that can be sterilized periodically by boiling. Salespeople can show you the various systems if you ask. External drainage works well for many men who do not self-cath. Some use external drainage only for special occasions when self-cath would be too much of a nuisance.

External drainage catheters have recently become available for women as well. I have no personal experience with their use, but several of my correspondents have begun to experiment with them. If you are interested in such an arrangement, speak with your local Physicians and Hospital Supply store, to inquire about available systems.

MANAGEMENT OF BLADDER SPASTICITY

Bladder spasticity is not as dangerous as bladder flaccidity. Bladder infection does not develop after repeated forcible bladder emptying.

Cystometrogram Diagnoses
Bladder Malfunction

The cystometrogram graphically demonstrates the dysfunction of a spastic bladder. (See discussion, page 319, and Fig. 17-4, page 320.) In this figure, uninhibited bladder spasms dominate both the cystometrogram and the bladder's owner once the residual urine volume is exceeded. Electrical evaluation of bladder neck muscles is often performed at the same time. If your urologist has equipment to do this part of the examination, you can learn whether your bladder neck also goes into spasm when the bladder wall contracts. In this case, Dibenzyline® may help to manage your urgency-hesitancy symptoms. (See page 121.) In some cases, bladder neck muscles relax involuntarily, causing sudden incontinence without urgency. If you have this troublesome symptom, regularly timed self-cath will prevent the bladder from filling completely, so the volume of incontinence is limited. Adult diapers can catch incontinence that does occur. The solution is inadequate, but I have found no better one. Do my readers have an answer?

Use of Ditropan® for Spastic Bladder

Ditropan® (oxybutynin chloride) and several related medications reduce smooth muscle spasms in the bladder and promote bladder filling. Learn to use one of these when you first develop spastic bladder symptoms. Do you avoid automobile trips because bouncing of the car causes bladder spasms and incontinence? Have you stopped going out for bridge because the bathroom is too far from the den? If bladder spasms restrict your freedom, they can be abolished. *Take just enough medication to stop the spasms while you are active, without causing constant bladder flaccidity through chronic overdosage.*

I have used Ditropan exclusively for many years, but if your physician prefers one of the other preparations, use it and consider the guidelines for Ditropan. The goal of treatment is the same: A bladder that has no spasms during the active day, but returns to its spastic state at least once a day, so it can empty completely.

Strategy for Use of Ditropan

Most MSers first take a single dose of Ditropan for a special occasion. While Ditropan is active, spasms are eliminated, but it should still be possible to urinate from a filled bladder. After three to 10 hours, bladder spasms return with increasing urgency. That is the time to empty the bladder completely.

For those whose spasticity becomes a chronic nuisance, Ditropan can relieve it permanently. Urinate each morning and empty the bladder as completely as possible. Then use a dose of Ditropan large enough to prevent spasms during the day but not so large that it keeps the bladder flaccid through the evening. Most people use one or two tablets each morning.

Be *certain* that your bladder returns to its old spastic state by suppertime or early evening before you even *think* of taking another dose! If bladder spasms disturb nighttime sleep, take a dose before going to bed. This will control spasms till morning.

This advice differs from the package insert. It recommends one tablet three or four times a day without considering the state of bladder function. As a result of this repetitive dosage schedule, the bladder may develop constant flaccidity. When that happens, frequency and urgency return because the flaccid bladder has enlarged to its fullest capacity. This feels just like the frequency and urgency before Ditropan and can confuse the MSer who is unaware of the possibility. Worse yet, constant flaccidity encourages the development of bladder infections.

Use Ditropan, to decrease bladder spasticity during most of the day and most of the night. Accept the idea that your bladder must return to its old nasty spastic state at least once a day, so it can empty as completely as possible. As you begin, take Ditropan once in the morning and note the duration of action. To discover your proper dose, try one tablet on the morning of the first two days. Note the effect on bladder function. Take two tablets on the third and fourth days and note the effect.

The usual dose is one or two tablets. Do not take more than two doses in 24 hours. You will know by the fourth day which dose works best for you. If you have an important appointment during the day, take an extra dose to get through without embarrassment. Next day be certain that your bladder has recovered, or you will end up with a flaccid bladder.

If it seems to you that Ditropan has stopped working, stop the medication completely for several days. If you already know self-cath, test yourself for bladder enlargement and then, through repeated self-cath, document its return to normal.

Warnings About Use of Ditropan®

Most MSers can use Ditropan successfully, but there are some contraindications.

If you have glaucoma, never use Ditropan. It can increase already elevated pressure in the eye, causing progressive visual loss, that could be mistaken for optic neuritis.

Ditropan may aggravate esophageal irritation (from hiatus hernia), and also ulcerative colitis.

Prostatic enlargement itself may cause urinary retention, *without* medication. Ditropan can worsen that tendency by causing decreased contractility of the bladder wall.

Ditropan can interfere with sweating. In summertime take extra precautions to be certain your body temperature stays normal, so the heat does not affect you unnecessarily.

Any MSer unfortunate enough to have myasthenia gravis as well, should avoid Ditropan.

There is no accurate information about the effects of Ditropan on the developing fetus. However, pregnant women should avoid Ditropan, and other medications if possible, during at least the first four months of pregnancy.

MANAGEMENT OF URGENCY WITH SEVERE HESITANCY

Spastic legs tire easily and refuse to walk properly on command. Spastic bladders never tire, but often refuse to urinate on command. As the normal bladder wall *contracts* to begin urination, muscles at the bladder neck *relax*, allowing urine to leave the bladder and enter the urethra. In MS bladders, the muscles around the bladder neck may forget to relax when they should, obstructing the flow of urine at the very moment of worst urgency. It may take 20 minutes of waiting and trying before the bladder neck muscle finally relaxes and urination can occur. This is called detrusor-sphincter dyssynergia ("bladder *wall* muscle—bladder *neck* muscle incoordination"). The dyssynergia disrupts a pleasant day. It is dysagreeable, dysadvantageous and dyscouraging. It makes MSers dysconsolate, dysgruntled and dyscommoded. It is a major nuisance.

The cause of detrusor-sphincter dyssynergia is spasm of muscles at the bladder neck. Recent investigations have shown that these muscles respond specifically to medications like Dibenzyline® , (phenoxybenzamine) or its chemical relatives, which block one type of autonomic innervation. A dose of 10 mg. up to four times a day, promotes bladder emptying. Dibenzyline prevents spasm of bladder neck muscles, decreases hesitancy, improves urinary stream and helps to reduce residual urine volume. The major symptom is tremendous urgency, coupled with inability to urinate. Seek the cause by requesting urodynamic studies. (See page 319.) If such studies are hard to arrange, ask for a prescription for Dibenzyline to determine whether it can provide relief.

The major side effect of Dibenzyline is dizziness, sometimes worsened by getting up from sitting or lying down. As we have mentioned for other medications, pregnant women should avoid Dibenzyline and other medications, because their effect on the developing fetus is unknown.

HOW WILL I KNOW TO CHANGE FROM SPASTICITY MANAGMENT TO FLACCIDITY MANAGEMENT?

I have trouble advising MSers as they emerge from successful management of a spastic bladder, and discover to their dismay that this week Ditropan makes things worse. My first assumption is that the bladder is overdosed, so we stop the pills. This usually improves bladder function. If the bladder has become more flaccid, a limited use of Ditropan several days later may again cause incontinence.

For MSers who know self-cath, the problem is easier. When Ditropan fails, we check the residual urine volume immediately. If the person has kept records, we then know how the residual urine volume has changed. Usually we stop Ditropan and return to self-cath. Once the residual falls again, Ditropan might again be useful. If Ditropan failed because MS caused more bladder flaccidity, it cannot again be the sole mode of management until MS again adds spasticity to bladder function.

How will I Find a Toilet once I Know all this?

"The question isn't so much bladder control, as where to find accessible toilets," wrote one of our editors, as she went through this chapter.

122

"All of your suggestions for management are fine, but the most pressing question remains: When I go out to lunch with friends, where is the accessible toilet where I can use all those nice management techniques? Don't tell me to go before I leave. My bladder has a mind of its own, and it *knows* when there is no accessible toilet."

Now there's a problem! Steve Fellows pointed out in his chapter that a governmental agency's definition of accessible may be different from the MSer's. Restaurants may be even flightier about their definitions. Do my readers know? Do they keep a list of local accessible establishments for junior people to use and update? Do some local agencies keep such a file? Do you want to start one?

Perhaps you want to use a trick that MSers in Syracuse use. They take a coffee can with them, complete with plastic top. It can be used in the car, in a tent, at an inaccessible toilet, or even under the table at a posh restaurant. Seal the lid and contents after use, and dump it at your leisure.

INDWELLING CATHETER DRAINAGE

If none of the foregoing techniques works, and diapers smell or have caused skin breakdown, an indwelling catheter is a good solution to a bad problem. Once the catheter is in place, incontinence stops. The bed and skin around the bottom remain dry. Odor disappears. The catheter frees you from bladder worries so you can move on to more interesting problems. Even the washing machine gets a rest.

There are also disadvantages. Once the indwelling

123

catheter is inserted, the bladder shrinks around it to a very small size. If indwelling catheterization is used briefly, but for more than a day or two, follow these precautions: Clamp it continuously to allow the bladder to fill, then open the clamp briefly every two to six hours when it is full, to allow it to drain. This tidal technique prevents bladder shrinkage and promotes rapid return to more normal function.

Temporary indwelling catheterization may be extremely useful for the MSer who cannot plan to self-cath for a day. Is your daughter graduating from college this weekend? Use your self-cath skills to insert a 16 French Foley catheter with a 5 cc bulb. Leave it in place during the endless ceremonies until the exciting part when she has the spotlight. While other parents squirm in discomfort, your leg bag will fill quietly. When you get home, remove the catheter, boil it, dry it, and put it away for the next occasion.

Choice of Catheter and Catheter Management

Use the smallest catheter that prevents urine from leaking around it. Most adults can start with a 16 Fr. Foley catheter with a five cc. bulb. After months or years of continuous catheterization, the urethra enlarges and urine begins to leak around the catheter. When this happens, simply graduate to a catheter two to four Fr. larger. Use the green Silastic® catheters, not the tan rubber ones. Silastic sheds debris better so it does not plug up as fast as rubber. Always keep at least one spare in the house.

All catheters plug up eventually, but the interval may be increased by good management practices. Calcium salts and mucus are the chief enemies. Change of diet can minimize calcium build-up. Avoid large amounts of dairy products like milk, ice cream and cheese, because their calcium content is excreted in the urine and finds its way to your catheter. High daily urine flow and urine acidification help to prevent encrustation of the catheter tip. Bladder cleanliness is important.

You, and someone in the family, should know how to remove the catheter and replace it with a new one. Catheters have the bad habit of plugging up during the wee hours of a Sunday morning when no professional help is available. This dire emergency is completely preventable. If you and your family know what to do, do it and go about your business. If you do not, you must rush to the nearest emergency room for an expensive, tiring catheter change that could have been done at home.

How will you know when the catheter is plugged? After the first time, you will have no trouble recognizing it. There will be no urine in the night bag. Palpation of the abdomen reveals a hard, tender bladder. As bladder distension worsens, headache, fever and chills begin. Frantic attempts at bladder irrigation fail . . . .

. . . No problem! When the first symptoms of obstruction appear, remove the catheter, and replace it with a new one. If you don't yet know how to do it, learn now, before it plugs up again.

A professional will teach you to use sterile gloves and sterile technique for catheter changes. Despite the presence of bacteria in the bladder, it is wise to prevent new strains of bacteria from getting in and causing trouble. Use sterile technique.

Bladder Cleanliness

Keep your bladder clean. Acidify the urine with enough vitamin C to keep the pH below 6.5. Test it with pH paper or with Combistix® to keep the pH right. (See page 105.) Irrigate the bladder at least once a day, using a large bulb syringe. Fill the syringe with irrigation solution and inject the solution through the catheter into the bladder. Force it in vigorously and suck it out again completely. Discard each dose of irrigation solution when you have removed it. Do this repeatedly until the returns are clear and you have swished out all the bacteria, calcium flecks, mucus and gunk that have collected since last time. If you do this daily, it takes only a few minutes. If you neglect your bladder, the job takes forever.

Irrigation solution may be purchased, but it is expensive. Make your own irrigation solution for pennies at home. Use about two level tablespoons (30 cc.) of non-iodized salt per gallon of water. Boil for about 10 minutes to sterilize the solution. Allow it to cool to room temperature, then pour the solution into clean gallon containers. Add two or three *drops* of household vinegar per gallon. Too much vinegar will burn when you irrigate. Two drops per gallon provides a touch of acidity, and smells nice into the bargain. Gallon sherry bottles make excellent storage containers, and their original contents contributes to interesting conversation before bedtime.

Catheters and Sex

Some women avoid using the indwelling catheter because they are concerned that sexual intercourse would be forbidden. This is not so. Although sexual intercourse adds one more risk of infection to the list already enumerated, it does not *automatically* lead to infection. Nor does abstinence automatically protect against it. If you decide that an indwelling catheter would solve problems of bladder malfunction, use it and continue to have intercourse. In any event, maintain an excellent bladder regimen.

Some couples decide to remove the catheter each time they have sex. Others simply pull it to one side or tape it to the abdomen. Removal and reinsertion carry slightly more risk, but if you find it more attractive despite the nuisance, do what feels right.

SUMMARY

Successful MSers develop a combination of management techniques that help them adjust to change. This requires vigilance and occasional reassessment of bladder function. If you develop expertise, you may be able to do most of this at home. Actually, the process is not as hard as it sounds. A limited number of techniques encompass all of bladder management. If you have trouble deciding how to combine these techniques and to apply them to your changing bladder function, this chapter may offer some helpful ideas. Keep a record of successes and failures. Learn from your doctor, from other MSers and from your previous experience. Teach junior MSers coming up behind you. Keep the professionals in your life informed. Keep trying. Your aggressive decision to take charge will be more important to you than any words from me. That decision and your actions can improve your life in future years.

Master the few techniques of bladder management we have discussed so you can continue your life without losing your urine or your composure. You can prevent most infections. You can avoid or manage almost all emergencies. Individual procedures sound hard, but once they have been mastered they are straightforward and simple.

Choose proper management over complications. Persevere through hard times, because excellent bladder management for the rest of your life is worth far more than the limited effort you invest.

Chapter 6
Bowel Control
By John K. Wolf

No one can be assured of perfect bowel control. But *almost* all the time, MSers can have bowel movements on schedule and avoid fecal incontinence. Happily, the techniques are much less complex than those used for bladder control.

MANAGEMENT OF EARLY SYMPTOMS

The complaint of constipation usually means that an MSer who once had a bowel movement every morning, now has it only once in two or three days. That is not constipation. Real constipation means that BMs refuse to move, or do so reluctantly. If the movements themselves are easy, ready when you are, and not incontinent, they are normal—even if they occur only once in 10 days.

Everyone spends time thinking about bowel function, and so will you. Devise a dietary regimen that produces formed but pliable stools. Instead of using laxatives that irritate the bowel, eat enough roughage to fill the rectum every day or every other day so you can empty it on schedule and at your command. Avoid water restriction and diuretics if possible.

If these simple means work, move on to the next chapter. If not, think about these questions: Have you had just one episode of fecal impaction that required professional help? Are your bowels usually difficult to move? Have you been incontinent just once? If you answer yes to any of these questions, you may want to spend more time planning your bowel regimen. The time and effort spent, plus your change in attitude, will result in improved regularity and diminished anxiety.

Once you make that decision, your attitude toward food may change: That delicious beefsteak, salad and bran muffin doused in honey will become raw material for a product!

Common Causes of Real Constipation

Reduced physical activity causes constipation. This happens among physically healthy people with the flu, or during a hospital admission for surgery. MSers are forced into reduced physical activity. They may also have abnormal bowel innervation, so they are even more likely to have trouble. The solution? ... A well-planned diet.

MSers who limit daily fluid intake in a mistaken attempt to control bladder function, find that the body conserves water where it finds it. The colon sucks water out of the feces, changing nice soft, fluffy stool into hard, inflexible globs like the ones illustrated in Fig. 6-1.

Meat and potatoes contain no bulk once they arrive in the colon. Unless accompanied by roughage, the result is highly concentrated, hard stool that can't pass through the anus. Those who eat less to retain slim lines may neglect to eat enough salads, vegetables and cereals. A diet poor in roughage produces a firm, concentrated stool. The colon has a larger diameter than the rectum, and the muscle around the anus is even smaller. Hard, inflexible globs will not pass through the anus, and may even get stuck above the rectum.

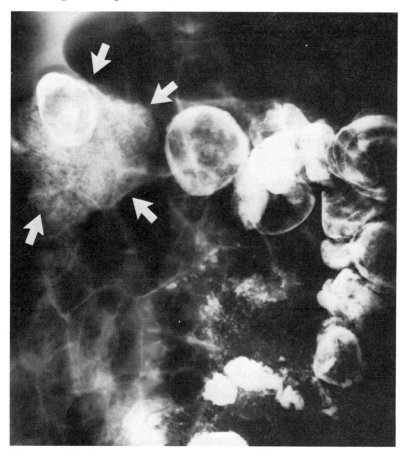

Fig. 6-1. Fecal impaction outlined by barium contrast. The barium was injected under the mistaken impression that three days of enemas had cleared the colon. Only the rectum is partially cleared (lower right). Most of the colon is still filled with hard inflexible stool. The soft stool (arrows upper left) in the first part of the colon cannot possibly pass unless the rest is first expelled by repeated saline enemas. Careful attention to diet prevents this complication.

You Probably Do Not Need Laxatives

Laxatives like Metamucil® (psyllium hydrophilic muciloid) increase fecal bulk. Colace® and related compounds contain dioctyl sodium sulfosuccinate which softens and moistens the stool. Some laxatives irritate the bowel wall and cause it to produce mucus and increased colonic contractions. This class of laxative often leaves an irritated, dripping rectum that embarrasses its owner for hours after the BM.

A rectum filled with soft but formed stool is ready to go and will usually empty on command. A half-filled rectum may refuse to move in the morning, but fills later in the day to produce an urgent need or actual incontinence. Liquid stool is incontinent if the anal muscle is imperfect. Avoid liquid stools at all cost.

You may use prescription laxatives if you like, but I prefer bran. You should not need a doctor or a pharmacist to have a bowel movement. Bran is available at the grocery store. It comes in delicious cereals for breakfast. It may be incorporated into muffins, bread and even meatloaf for lunch and supper. Bran works, and bran is predictable. Too predictable. I know.

Almost 10 years ago, my family and I drove to Florida from Syracuse to visit my parents. I discovered bran on that trip. I planned to drive through the night while the family slept, in order to put as many miles as possible behind us. On the afternoon of our departure I bought snacks to keep me awake and my stomach comfy during the long night's drive: Crackers, cheddar cheese, candy and two boxes of a cereal I had never before seen, called "Cracklin' Bran."

We left home after supper and I began to munch before midnight. I opened the "Cracklin' Bran" and discovered scrumptious little doughnuts of bran and brown sugar which left an aftertaste that asked for more. I ate only a little of the cheese and crackers, never touched the candy, but downed a box and a half of those delicious little bran doughnuts before early morning. When we reached the beltline around Washington, D.C., we stopped at a gas station. I then lay down to sleep while Mitzi drove on.

"Funny," I thought about an hour later, "I thought I just *did* that!"

But we stopped again—and again—and yet again, all day long, compensating for our initial good start by taking sightseeing trips to rest stops, roadside woods and many other places that interested only me, while my family smiled behind their hands. I *know* about Cracklin' Bran but I have never used it properly. Whenever Mitzi brings it home, I O.D. on it because it is so good. Others are more successful.

There is a Better Way

Taken daily, the right amount of bran dramatically changes the bulk and consistency of the stool. A proper dose fills the rectum on schedule with light, fluffy, soft stool that is ready to go. Too large a dose fills it by midnight. Very large doses fill it regularly on the hour for as long as you like—longer, even.

Begin small. Increase the amount of bran you use by a couple of spoonsful every three or four days. Observe the result before you move to the next dosage level. You have had your bowels for many years, so there is no need to have instant familiarity with bran. If you begin slowly and in a controlled manner, you will discover the proper dose without trouble. Most people need a bowl or two each day, but some need only a few spoonsful. If you rush right in, you may find yourself stopping by woods on a snowy evening, when you would prefer to be home in bed. Bran will work you, never fear. But determine your dose carefully.

Remember the Rest of Your Diet, Too

As you experiment with bran, consider also the effect of the rest of your diet on your bowel movements. If your diet is not approximately the same from day to day, you may have to deal with a sudden surge of roughage from that Caesar salad you ate last night along with the usual portion of bran. Be aware of the interrelationship of bran and your daily diet. Vary each accordingly. Begin slowly. Change the amount of bran with care. Observe the results and you will succeed.

The discussion of bran in our first edition prompted a letter from an old friend, a retired physician. He told of a man who regularly made a *Gemisch* of diced prunes, figs and raisins. After mixing, he formed these into a loaf which he kept in the refrigerator. When he felt the need, he broke off a chunk of his "cr—— cake," and found this a satisfying remedy to a common problem.

MANAGEMENT OF MORE SEVERE BOWEL DYSFUNCTION

Early control measures become inadequate as MS becomes more advanced. An empty rectum cannot become incontinent, so *scheduled and regular emptying* is the goal of management. There are ways to assure an empty rectum for most of the day, and so prevent incontinence.

The Gastro-Colic Reflex

Honey and lemon juice in boiling water kept my father-in-law, Fred Beisswenger, regular. For years he promoted his concoction to me, even though I had no need of it. He is dead now, but I have taken up the campaign. Hot coffee or tea also stimulate the gastro-colic reflex.

When warm food or drink enters the stomach, this reflex starts contractions in the colon which move its contents into the rectum and and prepare for a BM. You learned that lesson when your babies needed a diaper change only minutes after each bottle. We have become accustomed to suppressing the reflex in our busy lives. Now you can re-educate your bowel, and use the reflex to good advantage.

Begin your day with a hot drink. Wait 30 minutes to allow the gastro-colic reflex time to work. Then bring the morning paper or *Time Magazine* with you into the bathroom.

Local Sacral Reflexes

Several MSers have found they could start a BM by scratching the skin between the buttocks just above the anus. This skin is innervated from the same sacral spinal cord segments as the rectum and anus. Scratching of the skin seems to activate a local reflex that stimulates rectal contractions and helps to start the movement. If the gastro-colic reflex alone fails, scratch between the buttocks and hold *Time* with only one hand.

Suppositories

Suppositories cause a BM both by increasing rectal gland secretion and by stimulating rectal contractions. The result is a bowel movement that would otherwise have waited. Be careful with suppositories. The highly potent ones irritate the rectum so severely that they overpower a careful regimen of bowel control and empty the entire colon in a single spasm. Potent suppositories are a prescription item. They are unnecessary for routine bowel management, and can cause distinctly undesirable side effects later in the day, like further dripping, spasms and incontinence.

Glycerine suppositories are far less irritating and are available over the counter. You used them for your babies and you can use them now for yourself. Glycerine also stimulates the rectal lining and causes increased rectal contractions, but the stimulus is milder. If the rectum is filled with soft, fluffy stool, a glycerine suppository helps to produce a BM on demand.

Drink your honey and lemon juice in hot water. Wait 30 minutes. Insert a glycerine suppository three quarters of the way into the rectum, and leave enough protruding so you can get it out again in 30 minutes if no BM occurs. Do not leave the suppository in place if you have no BM this time. It will continue to irritate and probably will cause later incontinence. I don't know what you did with *Time* this trip, but I hope you enjoyed it!

The Problem Revisited

In the first edition, editor Barbara Shetron raised a vital question about glycerine suppositories, which remains unanswered to this day.

> "How do numb, uncoordinated fingers hold
> onto those slippery little beggars?"

She uses them infrequently because five out of six end up in the toilet bowl. My editors had no answer. I suggested several inadequate solutions. Only Bonnie Johannes, has offered an improvement.

"Eureka! (well, maybe) It occurred to me as I lay on my side in bed reading, that instead of inserting the suppository on the toilet sitting up, why not insert it lying in that position? That way, dropped suppositories can be found and rescued, rather than lost! Maybe a cotton glove would hold the suppository without slippage. —Or the rubber finger tips and thumb tips secretaries use, to count through lots of papers."

In several places I have asked for readers' help with unsolved problems. Bonnie is agile enough to get to the toilet before the thing begins to work. She is also agile of mind. In addition to the gloves and finger tips, she devised a picture of a "suppository syringe" with markings on it to indicate when the suppository is in proper position. It is a beginning. But the elusive perfect solution is still out there somewhere. The field remains open for competition.

Vaginal Pressure

Women have the advantage over men because the back wall of the vagina is immediately adjacent to the front wall of the rectum. A finger in the vagina, pressing downward and backward, can move stool that otherwise might have stuck. Such pressure also straightens the rectum to a more vertical position, so the usual technique, "take a deep breath and push," empties more easily.

Direct Anal Stimulation

I had not known how useful direct anal stimulation could be until Dr. Arthur Ecker called my attention to it. Since then I have found MSers who don a finger cot (a rubber finger "glove") to dilate the anus and start a movement.

Try using a rectal syringe (or a bulb syringe) to dilate the anus. These are easily available at your local physicians and hospital supply store. Inject water above the first piece, especially if there is a hard unwilling stool barring the exit. Use of bran from that day forward might prevent a return of the problem.

Enemas

Almost everyone can devise a bowel regimen to fill the rectum regularly with soft, pliable stool. Occasionally, even the best regimens fail. The resulting fecal impaction is too tight to remove by simple means. You must know how to give yourself an enema, or have a family member who can do it with you. The most common cause of fecal impaction? You already know. Dietary mistakes: lack of bulk or adequate fluid intake.

Warning! The first sign of a fecal impaction may be intermittent diarrhea. Do not reach for the Kaopectate® at the first sign of diarrhea. Think first: When was the last good bowel movement? Have I been due for several days without result? Put on a glove or finger cot and feel inside the rectum. Is there a hard inflexible glob? If there is, clear the bowel with an enema and start again.

Fleet's® enemas come prepackaged and ready to use. This is the ideal disposable package for the MSer who needs enemas only occasionally. It can be stored till needed, and is highly effective. The emptied container may be refilled with water and used again at some later time.

Recipe for Enema Solution

If you need enemas frequently, buy a reusable enema bag and become an expert. Enema solution is easy to make. Warm tap water is often sufficient. If you like lubrication in your enemas, add a tablespoonful or so of castile soap, but be careful not to make foam when you add it. If yours is a difficult impaction requiring more than one infusion, do not use plain tap water. It could suck needed salts from the blood stream through the bowel wall. Instead, use the saline solution described on page 126 for bladder irrigation, but *without* the vinegar.

Enema Technique

The technique is simple. Add about a quart of warm tap water or enema solution of your choice to the enema bag. Hang on a rod or hook, out of the way, but above the target. Fasten the clip so no solution can flow out of the bag till you are ready. Lubricate the end of the tube with water soluble lubricating jelly and insert the tube as far as it will go without resistance. Do not force the tube past obstructions. You may be pushing directly on the bowel wall instead of on feces and do yourself damage.

If you can, take your enemas on the toilet or commode. It is much less messy this way. If that is too difficult, line the bed with Chux®, newspapers, or a plastic sheet to catch water and debris. Then sit on a regular bedpan. Do not use the more comfortable fracture pan for an enema, because its small capacity will cause an overflow. If you need help, lie on your back, knees separated and bent so the operator has free access to the anus.

Plan to hold all the solution you can. Release the clip and allow solution to flow. If it begins to leak out, stop the flow for a few moments and try again. When you find you have taken all your rectum can hold—wait. The action will begin in a minute. Women can help by pushing backward and downward on the back wall of the vagina. Take a deep breath and push—*slowly, or you will have a gusher!* Once fluid and stool have been ejected, wait a few more minutes. There may be more above. Because you never can be certain how many infusions you will need, it is an excellent plan always to use the saline enema solution, with or without castile soap.

Do not use enemas more frequently than every five to seven days. If the enema empties the entire colon, no BM is *possible* until the colon fills again. Follow a better dietary regimen and wait for it to fill the colon with moist pliable, bran-filled, fluffy stool. At day four or five, try the usual effective procedures. Use the gastro-colic reflex. Scratch between the buttocks. Discover a good way to hold a glycerine suppository—and tell the rest of us your technique. Read *Time Magazine* carefully from cover to cover and learn from Dr. Edward Fingl, who wrote in the Sixth Edition of Goodman and Gilman's *Pharmacological Basis of Therapeutics* that "haste does not make waste." You may even have to wait a day or two and try again each day before your rectum is ready. Don't rush back to the enema bag until you know you need it.

Manual Disimpaction

MSers sometimes decide that weekly manual disimpaction is preferable to messy BMs in bed. They prefer to eat what they please and allow hard, inflexible stool to accumulate, which is never incontinent. They opt for a weekly manual disimpaction.

This is not a bad plan if all else fails. Family members can learn to do manual disimpaction. Before you plan such a program, be certain that your family really wants to do this for you. If they do, and if you can accept their personal care, ask the Visiting Nurse to teach them. If your family prefers not to give you enemas, hire a professional on a regular basis. In any event, prepare enema solution, and store it in another set of emptied gallon sherry jugs. Plan to enjoy *scintillating* conversations before bedtime while preparing the containers for their new job. For easy distinction between bladder solution and enema solution, your author suggests purchasing two different brands of sherry!

SUMMARY

There you have it. Decide on your goals for bowel management and work constantly toward those goals:

1) Bowel movements will occur on a regular schedule.

2) They will *never* (well, hardly ever) occur by accident.

3) Stool will be formed, but soft enough to pass through the anus from the rectum. Diarrhea will be avoided at all cost.

4) As much as possible, prescription drugs, strong laxatives and mechanical procedures like enemas will be avoided.

Do everything you must to achieve these goals. Never stop striving for perfection. Effective management plans for bowel control, like effective management for every other symptom, allow you to proceed more confidently with your life, and to be a more effective person, regardless of the degree of your disability.

ATTENTION!

Please read the description of Prozac on page 212. This new, highly effective antidepressant, should also be considered in treatment of MS depression.

Chapter 7

Diagnosis and Management of Depression
By John K. Wolf

A death in the family, unpaid bills, the recent diagnosis of MS: these are universally depressing. Normal depression is a response to a real situation. It improves with time, as the person learns to cope. We all weep from time to time, but after a good cry, we pull ourselves together and go forward.

A sad event may trigger MS depression, but instead of improving with time, it lingers. It destroys joy and interrupts the flow of life from within. Irritability and querulous behavior disrupt family harmony. Both sufferer and family may fail to recognize depression because there is no reason for it. Even after identifying it, they often cannot combat it.

If you recognize yourself or a family member as you read this chapter, talk with your doctor about it. An accurate diagnosis of depression can lead to effective treatment that will help you return to the land of the living.

A PICTURE OF DEPRESSION

Socks dumped on the floor are an annoyance to anyone, but to the depressed person they become a symbol of the family's indifference, lack of love, or downright hatefulness. Instead of the crisp command, "Pick up your socks!" there is an outburst of anger and recrimination. During depressed outbursts, MSers are sometimes so upset that they strike out violently against anyone or anything within reach. The little things that trigger the blow-up are real, but the response is out of proportion to the event.

Depressed weeping is different from normal weeping. When it finally stops, it leaves no comfort. Like depressed anger, depressed weeping begins with little or no cause. Instead of stopping after a few minutes, depressed weeping continues for half an hour or more, and seems to have a life of its own. Depressed MSers sometimes weep when they are not sad, and weeping continues long after they are ready to stop.

Sleep suffers. Depressed people fall asleep when they retire, but they wake in the night to spend many hours tossing and turning. They feel alone and uncared-for. They rehash unhappy events from the recent and distant past that are relevant only to the depression. Sleepless nights increase fatigue. Dishes pile up in the sink. The house is cluttered. Office work remains unfinished. Extra activities are abandoned for lack of energy.

Body posture changes. The shoulders sag. Gait is slowed and shuffling. The face and voice are sad even when the person smiles. The voice loses its normal quality. Its tone becomes flat and uninteresting. Sad sighs punctuate waking hours. Even casual conversations are burdensome. Personal relationships at home and at work deteriorate. Reclusiveness becomes a way of life. Terrible! These changes are difficult to describe, but once recognized, they are unmistakable.

The problem is, usually no one knows! We expect others to pull their weight at home and at work. We resent unjustified anger and irrational weeping. When someone changes so completely because of unrecognized depression, the angry reactions of friends and family only make things worse.

This kind of depression is so common among MSers, that it is now recognized as a specific symptom of MS (1,4)*. Although MS depression can be terrible, it is usually not as severe as I have portrayed it. Fortunately, once recognized, it is treatable.

TREATMENT OF DEPRESSION

The insidious depression of MS responds well to treatment. Antidepressant medications should be given to the MSer whose life is disrupted by depression and who is willing to take antidepressants.

Unfortunately, some MSers are unwilling to take antidepressant medications because of the social stigma of any ''psychiatric'' diagnosis. If you recognize yourself in this chapter but have that lingering prejudice, please re-think your priorities. Are you more interested in avoiding the diagnosis of a treatable symptom of MS than in returning to your life?

Table 7-1 lists the antidepressants available in the United States. Physicians are usually acquainted with

---

* Note: References for this chapter may be found on page 157.

one or more of them, and employ them with some regularity. Each has side effects. Some may have a more rapid onset of action. Some cause more sedation. Others more dryness of the mouth. All are effective in treatment of some people with depression. You and your doctor must work together to find which one is best for you.

My own preferred antidepressant for MSers is Elavil® (amitriptyline). It causes more initial sleepiness than some of the others, but after months of insomnia, five good nights of rest are a blessing. Elavil causes one lasting side effect: dry mouth. Not to worry. Drink more water. If you have read the chapters on bowel and bladder management, you already know that increased water intake is a definite benefit.

The major disadvantage of Elavil is its long biological half-life. (See page 87.) Elavil accumulates in the body for about two weeks before its concentration becomes stable. If the first dose is too small to combat depression, wait two weeks before increasing the dose, and perhaps two weeks more before depression begins to clear. This is a serious disadvantage when treating severe psychotic depression. Fortunately, MSers do not usually have psychotic depression, so they can afford the wait. I like Elavil but prescribe the less expensive generic form.

Other treatments for depression are available, but are usually unnecessary. They should be taken only under the close supervision of a psychiatrist. Monoamine oxidase inhibitors fall into this category. Lithium carbonate has great value under specifically defined conditions. Phenothiazines and other major tranquilizers are good for treatment of psychosis, but if yours is the usual MSer depression, you do not need tranquilizers. Electroshock therapy is used only by psychiatrists.

Avoid using the minor tranquilizers like Valium®
(diazepam) and Librium® (chlordiazepoxide), which
have been prescribed indiscriminately in the past.
These are antianxiety agents, and may actually make
depression worse. Since depressed MSers respond so
well to Elavil, these other treatments are usually unnecessary.

When compared to Elavil, the "talking treatment"
and simple reassurance are ineffective. MS depression
is not caused by disordered life experiences. It is primarily the result of MS plaques somewhere in the depths of
the brain. The biochemical pathology of depression is
becoming better understood. Antidepressant medications attack that pathology. If you are depressed, get
medicinal treatment first. Once your thoughts have
cleared, go for counseling if you like, with a brain that's
eager to learn new things.

STRATEGY FOR TREATMENT WITH
ANTIDEPRESSANT MEDICATIONS

Here are a few rules for use of antidepressants. They
are determined by the biological half-life of the medications, by their effective dose and by the usual duration
of depression after treatment has begun.

The First Few Weeks of Treatment

1) *Take the daily dose at bedtime.* Because of their long
biological half-life (See page 87.), antidepressants accumulate and disappear slowly in the body. A single dose
per day is just as effective, and it is easier to remember.
The major early side effect is sleepiness, so use the side
effect to your advantage. Take your pills at bedtime and
get some rest!

2) *Begin with the standard starting dose,* which rarely produces incapacitating sleepiness or other side effects. The standard starting dose of Elavil, 75 mg. at bedtime, is usually inadequate to treat depression. In practice, nearly everyone with MS depression requires 100—125 mg. of Elavil each day. Some people need 150 mg. A few MSers need more.

Elavil comes in 10 mg. tablets as well as larger dosage forms. Physicians unfamiliar with its use often make the mistake of prescribing the 10 mg. tablets and suggesting a total daily dose of 20—40 mg. This is inadequate to treat depression. Refer your physician to the *Physician's Desk Reference,* and ask to start at the standard starting dose, 75 mg. at bedtime.

Some people complain of uncomfortable sleepiness, even on the standard starting dose. If this happens to you, decrease the dose (if you are using Elavil) to 50 mg. per day for a week. Once your body has adjusted to the medication, go back to 75 mg. at bedtime. The effective dose is usually the same, despite early side effects. Plan to increase your total dose to 100—150 mg. per day as other people do, but more slowly.

3) Once you reach any dose, remember the long biological half-life and *wait the required period of time* (See table 7-1.) before increasing the dose. Usually it takes two weeks for blood and tissue concentrations to stabilize, so do not decide about your clinical response for at least two weeks. Then ask the specific questions that tell whether this is the right dose: Is there a distinct change in mood? Have weeping spells and anger outbursts stopped? Are you back to normal, slightly improved, unchanged?

The waiting period is critical. When I first learned to use Elavil, two of my patients called me in panic because I had not stressed the waiting period. They had increased their dose too fast, had arrived at too big a dose and now they had—the giggles! This felt just as abnormal and just as uncomfortable as depression. None of my arguments convinced either of them to reduce the dose and try again. I was inexperienced in giving instructions, so I lost the benefits of treatment for these two people. Avoid that mistake.

4) If there is no change, or only a slight change in mood after two weeks, *raise the dose by one dosage increment.* Use Table 7-1 as your guide to dosage increments. Do not make the mistake of accepting minimal improvement. Increase the dose deliberately till mood returns to normal. As you proceed, keep your doctor informed about your dose and your mood to get the best possible guidance in your search for your "best dose."

5) *Families often know before the MSer does, when the right dose has been reached.* Behavior changes dramatically when blood and tissue concentrations reach a therapeutic level. But even after depressed *behavior* has ended, depressed *thoughts* linger.

Two weeks after a depressed MSer has reached a proper dose, the family is enthusiastic. The voice has returned to normal. Temper outbursts and weeping spells have ceased. Sleep is restful and there is no more night time wandering. The family may have noticed a slight change on the previous dose and wondered whether this was adequate. Now they *know* they are on the right track.

The MSer, whose depressed thoughts still churn despite the improved mood, reports "no change."

"That's a lousy medicine, Doc. I feel just as

bad as I ever did, and you gave me a dry mouth too!''

Thoughts are still depressed. The person may still be mulling over inconsequential events from the past but does not recognize that these thoughts are no longer accompanied by the temper tantrums and weepiness of a few weeks past. It often takes another two to six weeks before the MSer realizes that depression has disappeared.

It is important to remember the delay between improved behavior and improved thought. The family is the first to know when the dose is right. They are the only accurate barometer of future blue skies or storm clouds.

And conversely, when the MSer stops the pills, family members notice immediately the return of depressed voice and posture. They recognize a temper tantrum without due cause, and they sense the return of other depressed behavior, banished by medication. These changes often occur before the MSer notices the return of depressed thoughts.

Strategy for Stopping Treatment

Plan with your family for your future use of antidepressants. Most people need antidepressant medications for six to 15 months, and can then stop without immediate return of depression. Knowing the usual duration of treatment, the MSer can agree to stay on the effective antidepressant dose for at least six months. After that time and *without telling anyone*, the MSer will begin to reduce the dose by one dosage increment (Table 7-1) each month. If the family barometers fail to recognize any change in behavior, then the dose is decreased again. If depression still does not return, the MSer can continue to reduce the medication monthly over a period of several months. Then, no longer depressed, the MSer can inform the family!

TABLE 9-1

Chemical	Product Name / Trade Name	Standard Daily Starting Dose	Therapeutic Dosage Range	Dosage Increments	Onset of Action	Wait Time Between Increments	How Supplied
Standard Tricyclic Antidepressants							
Imipramine	Generic avail. Tofranil SK-Pramine Presamine Imavate	75-100 mg.	75-300 mg.	25 mg.	7-14 days	2-3 weeks	Tablets 10, 25, 50 mg.
Amitriptyline	Generic avail. Elavil	75-100 mg.	75-200 mg.	25 mg.	7-14 days	2-3 weeks	Tablets 10, 25, 50, 75, 100 mg.
Desipramine	Norpramin Pertofrane	30-75 mg.	30-250 mg.	25 mg.	7-10 days	2-3 weeks	Tablets, Capsules 25, 50 mg.
Doxepin	Adapin Sinequan	75-100 mg.	75-250 mg.	25 mg.	14-21 days	4 weeks	Capsules 10, 25, 50, 100 mg. Liquid Concentrate 50 mg./5 cc. (tsp.)

Most people begin to decrease the dose before their depression is over, so it returns. At that time the family barometers will easily recognize the return of abnormal behavior and can ask:

TABLE 9-1 (Continued)

Nortriptyline	Aventyl	50-75 mg.	50-100 mg.	25 mg.	14-21 days	2-3 weeks	Capsules 25, 50 mg. Liquid Concentrate 50 mg./5 cc. (tsp.)
Protriptyline	Vivactil	10-15 mg.	15-60 mg.	5-10 mg.	7-14 days	2-3 weeks	Tablets 5, 10 mg.
Newer Antidepressants							
Maprotiline	Ludiomil	75-100 mg.	75-200 mg.	25 mg.	3-21 days	2-3 weeks	Tablets 25, 50 mg.
Amoxapine	Asendin	100-150 mg.	100-300 mg.	50 mg.	4-21 days	2-3 weeks	Tablets 50, 100, 150 mg.
Trazodone	Desyrel	100-150 mg.	100-400 mg.	50 mg.	4-21 days	2-3 weeks	Tablets 50, 100 mg.

The standard group of antidepressants are all tricyclic compounds with similar chemical structure. The newer antidepressants are chemically diverse. The possibility of a more rapid onset of action is an advantage, but all of them have delayed onset action in some people, so the waiting time between dosage increments is unchanged to guard against too rapid increase of dose among persons whose response *will* appear, but not at the accelerated time.

"Are you off your pills?"

The advantage of not telling is obvious. Had the family known in advance, they would have awaited the return of depressed behavior. If the MSer had scolded someone for throwing socks on the floor, they might accuse him of being depressed again.

Usually, depressed people do not accept first barometric reports that storm clouds loom on the horizon. After all, a temper tantrum may have occurred before depressed thoughts developed. An emotional outburst that sounds inappropriately violent to the family may not seem so to the person coming off medications. The job of the family is not to force the MSer back on pills, but to inform. Depressed people are not crazy. They are able to reason and think clearly, especially if they get feedback early in a depressed period. If family members have made an accurate diagnosis, the return of depressed thoughts, reappearance of weeping spells and temper tantrums convince most depressed people that the medication is needed. Once you make the decision, return to the proper dose, the same as it was before. Continue it for another four to six months and then try again.

Most people can finally stop treatment. Some stop periodically and go back again in six months or a year. Some must take Elavil for many years. If a medication makes life worth living, why not take it? Antidepressants are relatively safe for long-term use, and are preferable to the terrible disruptions caused by depression.

If You Live Alone

If you have no family, find a substitute barometer person. Do you have friends who visit regularly? Is there a nurse? Physical therapist? Clergyperson? Whoever sees you and knows you best can act as your barometer. Introduce them to the idea, to this chapter, and to your doctor, so all of you can be informed of your progress. Barometer people who are not immediate family may be a bit slower on the uptake, but they can help you to find the best antidepressant dosage.

Cautions About the Use of Antidepressants

Serious side effects are unusual, and the benefits of treatment are impressive. Most MSers appreciate Elavil or a related compound despite minor irritations like dry mouth and some sedation. Some MSers should investigate more serious complications, and talk with their physician before they accept treatment.

Glaucoma may suddenly flare up, causing pain and visual loss in one or both eyes. This complaint could be mistaken for optic neuritis! MSers with glaucoma must have their ocular pressures monitored as they use antidepressants. MSers on antidepressants who develop new visual complaints should remind the physician of this possible complication and ask for prompt referral for glaucoma testing.

Seizure disorder may become more difficult to control. Blood anticonvulsant levels should be checked before starting treatment and again soon afterward, to be certain they do not change. Kidney and liver disease may also be aggravated by antidepressants.

If you have heart failure, angina, disturbances of heart rhythm or have had a recent heart attack, speak to your doctor about using antidepressants. Such symptoms are serious contraindications to their use. Perhaps ask for help from a psychiatrist with experience in the use of these medications. Then decide if your depression warrants the risk. Fortunately, most MSers have normal hearts.

There is no accurate information about the effects of antidepressants on the developing fetus. Pregnant women should avoid antidepressants, and other medications if possible, during at least the first four months of pregnancy.

Emotional Incontinence is Not Depression

Some MSers and many other neurological patients have frequent brief episodes that are easily mistaken for depression. If someone unexpectedly walks into the room, if a brief sad remark is made, if the person laughs, a weeping spell may appear suddenly and without warning. Indeed, laughter may change directly into a weeping spell. The face is often contorted into a silent wail that resembles the worst of grief. The spells are brief, usually less than half a minute. Often there are no tears. When asked, the person says there is no accompanying sad emotion. Crying just happens. People are never violent during these attacks, and between spells, emotional tone is normal.

This is called "pseudobulbar emotionality" or "emotional incontinence." It occurs most commonly in people who have had bilateral stroke, but it can occur in *anyone* with lesions of *any* kind on both sides of the brain. I think of it as an accentuation of normal emotional responsiveness. When I listen to Puccini, for instance, I am not depressed. But his heartrending melodies, or merely Mimi's voice, always bring a catch to my breath and a lump to my throat that last throughout the performance.

After I have had my stroke or whatever, connections from my thinking brain to my feeling brain will be weakened and I won't be able to control my emotions as easily as I do now. Other people will see my emotional incontinence for the first time. I have been embarrassed by that response for years. The difference is, it never used to show.

Mike Sarette, one of our co-authors, described his own emotional incontinence. He sometimes becomes teary during M*A*S*H reruns or melodramatic sections of a novel. When something really serious happens, he reacts normally. He has discovered he can control the response if he takes a deep breath and concentrates on regular breathing. As they live with it, Mike and Bernice think his teariness is similar to spasticity. Short-circuited central control allows not anly a kneejerk, but also a tearjerk reaction.

Mike thinks that his response might be valuable to TV producers. They could hire MSers to identify their schmalziest sitcoms and improve their ratings!

Emotional Incontinence is Often Treatable

Emotional incontinence is sometimes controlled by levodopa, a medication with powerful effects on nerve cells deep in the brain. Levodopa is usually used against Parkinson's disease. Its effect on emotional incontinence was first noticed when emotional outbursts stopped for some Parkinson patients, even before there was improvement in their Parkinson symptons (5). A recent report has confirmed those original observations (3). If the description of easy laughing or crying in this section describes your situation, talk with your doctor about the use of levodopa. Begin with a small dose, 250 mg. three or four times a day, and increase the dose slowly at four to five day intervals to a maximum of 2000 mg. per day. If you choose the Sinemet® form of levodopa, begin with one 25/100 tablet three times a day and increase the dose by one tablet per day each week. The maximum dose of Sinemet is 5-6 tablets per day. If your easy laughing and crying do not stop on 2000 mg. per day of levodopa, or 5-6 of the 25/100 Sinemet® tablets, levodopa is ineffective for you and should be stopped.

Levodopa may cause nausea and sometimes vomiting. This can usually be controlled by taking it after meals or after a snack. Udaka's group (3) reports that amantadine also controls emotional incontinence for some patients. MSers who cannot use levodopa for some reason, should consider use of amantadine, 100 mg. once each day.

Low dose Elavil® may also be useful in suppressing emotional incontinence (2). The authors report dramatic cessation of inappropriate laughing and crying within two days of the start of treatment. They used lower doses than those needed for treatment of depression. Maximum was 75 mg. per day. Most patients needed less. Some of their patients failed to respond to Elavil, as some fail to respond to each of the other effective treatments described. If you do not respond to Elavil, try one of the other preparations indicated here.

There is no accurate information about the effects of levodopa, amantadine or Elavil on the developing fetus. Pregnant women should avoid these and other medications if possible, during at least the first four months of pregnancy.

REFERENCES:

1) Schiffer, R. B.; Babigian, H. M.: Behavioral Disorders in Multiple Sclerosis, Temporal Lobe Epilepsy, and Amyotrophic Lateral Sclerosis. *Arch. Neurol.* Vol. 41, Pages 1067–1069, 1984.

2) Schiffer, R. B.; Herndon, R. M.; Rudick, R. A.: Treatment of Pathologic Laughing and Weeping with Amitriptyline. *New England Journal of Medicine* Vol. 312, Pages 1480–1482, 1985.

3) Udaka, F.; Yamao, S.; Nagata, H.; Nakamura, S.; Kameyama, M.: Pathologic Laughing and Crying Treated with Levodopa. *Arch. Neurol.* Vol. 41, Pages 1095–1096, 1984.

4) Whitlock, F. A.; Siskind, M. M.: Depression as a Major Symptom of Multiple Sclerosis. *J. Neurol., Neurosurg., Psychiat.* Vol. 43, Pages 861–865, 1980.

5) Wolf, J. K.; Santana, H. B.; Thorpy, M.: Treatment of "Emotional Incontinence" with Levodopa. *Neurology* Vol. 29, Pages 1435–1436, 1979.

Chapter 8

The Pains of MS and their Management
By John K. Wolf

A rose without thorns is no rose.
Thorns without the flower are merely thorns.
But the two together, thorns and flower,
Are beauty.

Beauty without pain is superficial.
Pain without beauty is black.
But the two together, pain and beauty,
Are life!

Bonnie Johannes
May, 1983

"Why didn't you write anything about pain? I looked all through your book to find an explanation for mine, and there's nothing there!"

I have asked MSers to write in to complain, to suggest, to delete, to add. Jackie King and Betty Bistoff from the Syracuse area, and Lee Riley from Nashville, did. They are responsible for this chapter.

158

A chapter on pain would be first in a book on arthritis, but pain is a side issue in a book on MS. On the other hand, some MSers suffer considerable discomfort and pain during their lives. Most of it is treatable, so the pains of MS deserve discussion.

OPTIC NEURITIS

"When I woke up Tuesday morning I had a nagging, annoying pain in my right eye which worsened when I turned my eyes. By noon, vision in the eye was foggy. Colors appeared faded. Today I can't see to read, and the center of your face disappears when I look at you with that eye. The other eye is fine."

That is optic neuritis. Sometimes there is no pain. Sometimes pain occurs without much visual loss. Usually the pain is not excruciating, but it is often nasty and uncomfortable. It results from new MS damage to the optic nerve, which irritates the tissue immediately surrounding the nerve. A few days to two weeks after the inflammation has subsided and before vision returns, the pain disappears.

No treatment is required. Traditionally we prescribe prednisone or dexamethasone to relieve the pain of inflammation. Such medications taken during an attack of optic neuritis probably do not improve visual acuity over a lifetime, just as treatment for other acute exacerbations fails to change the long term course of MS. (See Chapters 10 and 19.)

Almost every MSer will eventually have optic neuritis. In Chapter 18 you will learn that visual evoked potential testing can provide evidence of previous optic neuritis in MSers who have never had visual symptoms.

There is a discussion of the anatomy of optic neuritis on page 311.

SPASTICITY

Diagnosis and management of spasticity is so important that we have devoted Chapter 4 to its management. When spasticity is painful, the pain usually responds to medications, physical therapy or physical support of weakened parts.

Weakness

Weakened muscles cannot support the body as they were meant to, so they work doubly hard. Activities that would be normal for physically healthy people are too taxing for spastic muscles and they react with pain.

Sometimes backache occurs for the same reason. Weakened leg and back muscles support the back poorly, resulting in stretched and painful ligaments. Treat these pains with heat and rest, but once you are rested, strengthen those muscles with physical therapy to keep the pain under better control. If the pain is unresponsive to routine pain medications, non-steroidal anti-inflammatory agents like Naprosyn® are occasionally useful.

Spastic Muscle Tightness

Tight spastic muscles hurt after exercise. In walking, normal muscles that control each joint relax and tighten alternately, to keep the body moving properly. Spastic muscles do not relax as they should. Instead, they pull against each other at every step. Spastic muscles aggravate exhaustion. They hurt after you walk, and ache in the evening after a day's activities. People with pain in spastic muscles know they have spasticity because of ankle clonus and spontaneous leg spasms. If you have this much spasticity and its resultant pains, read Chapter 4 and learn to use Lioresal®, or perhaps Dantrium®.

Painful Spastic Spasms

Painful spastic spasms result only from extremely severe and uncontrolled spasticity. At this stage the muscles are usually completely paralyzed for voluntary motion. They develop a life of their own and refuse to relax, causing severe pain. Lee Riley reports from Nashville, that her legs are most painful when both flexor and extensor muscles go into spasm at the same time. In all probability, you will not have painful spasms if you use Lioresal or Dantrium properly.

Shoulder Dislocation

Should you develop pain in a completely paralyzed shoulder, have it examined to determine if the weight of the arm has dislocated the shoulder joint downward. This is an uncommon complication of MS, but when it happens the pain can be managed, and contractures released, through heat and passive range of motion exercises. A sling may be used to support the elbow and forearm, so they no longer pull down against the shoulder ligaments.

LHERMITTE'S SIGN

"I get the strangest feeling when I bend my neck down!"

"Really? What's it like?"

"I can't explain it. It shoots down my left arm and down my back to my leg."

"Does it hurt?"

"Not exactly. It feels more like a shock or a tingle running down. The feeling disappears whether or not I lift my head again. Just a 'prrrrringgg!' and it's gone."

Lhermitte's sign is common among MSers. Lesions of many kinds in the cervical (neck) spinal cord can produce Lhermitte's sign, but it occurs mainly in MS.

The sensation is usually described as electrical, or tingling. It may shoot down the back to both legs, out one arm, down one side of the body. The distribution depends on the exact site of the lesion. It usually occurs when the neck is bent forward, but lasts only a moment. It then disappears whether or not the neck is straightened. Occasionally it remains as long as the neck is bent. One editor reported a continuous Lhermitte's sign, with or without movement.

Although it almost always comes from a plaque in the cervical spinal cord, I know one MSer whose Lhermitte's sign comes exclusively from lower segments. When she moves her trunk she gets the "prrrrringgg!" which starts at the right hipbone, and projects downward, almost to the knee, and upward as high as the the waist.

No treatment for Lhermitte's sign is available or necessary. Like other MS symptoms it comes and goes. It has no special significance for prognosis. It may be used in diagnosis as a definite sign that there is a lesion in the cervical spinal cord.

INFECTIONS CAUSE PAIN

Pain is one of the body's normal warning signals and should be observed carefully. Do you have pain on urination? Look for a bladder infection. (See Chapter 5, page 99–104.) Is there pain in your chest? Is it caused by pneumonia or bronchitis? Get an accurate diagnosis.

If you develop new pain, examine yourself to determine whether you need professional help. It is better sometimes to call when you *don't* need help rather than not to call when you really do.

SOME MS PAINS RESPOND TO TEGRETOL®, OTHER ANTICONVULSANTS, ELAVIL® , OR LIORESAL®

Tegretol® (carbamazepine) and Dilantin® (phenytoin) are primarily anticonvulsants. However, they also relieve certain pains arising in the nervous system. Most MSers never need Tegretol because their pain usually responds well to minor analgesics like aspirin, to Dilantin, or to antispastic medications like Lioresal. Occasionally, however, Tegretol is an excellent medication for relieving pain. But read also the warnings about Tegretol before you start to use it.

Tic Douloureux (Trigeminal Neuralgia)

Tic douloureux is an uncommon and extremely painful complication of MS. Because it is so rare, it is frequently misdiagnosed.

> "I have a terrible pain in my face!"
> "Really? Where is it?"
> "Right here in my cheek and upper jaw."
> "Must be a bad tooth. Let me look at it!"

But the pain of tic douloureux is different from the pain of a bad tooth. The distribution of the pain is limited by the anatomy of the trigeminal nerve. This nerve supplies sensation to the skin of the face, forehead and front of the scalp, to the insides of the cheeks and nasal passages, to teeth and gums and to the anterior two-thirds of the tongue. Tic douloureux usually occurs in only one division of the nerve's distribution, most commonly the second division which serves the inside and outside of the cheek, back across the face toward the ear, and the upper teeth.

The pain does not ache as an inflamed tooth does. You feel an extraordinarily intense burst of pain that lasts a second or two, occasionally followed by minutes of aching after-pain. A volley of painful shots may be set off by touching certain parts of the skin or the inside of the mouth. These areas are called "trigger points" and the sufferer may find it impossible to eat or shave without first touching the trigger point repeatedly to set off a series of tic pains. Thereafter, a brief pain-free interval occurs that allows the sufferer to do what needs to be done.

Tic douloureux is the only kind of pain an observer can actually see. The sufferer freezes suddenly in mid-sentence as the pain hits. There is perhaps a brief grunt of pain. If a series of shots occurs, everything stops until they have passed; thus the name, tic (sudden jerk) douloureux (caused by pain).

Tegretol usually stops the pain of tic douloureux. The pain often disappears after the first half-tablet and may be controlled throughout each 24 hours with repeated doses. Tic douloureux is one of the major indications for Tegretol. Do not fool around with aspirin for tic douloureux. Use Tegretol.

Sometimes, Tegretol alone is inadequate to stop tic pain. Fromm and Terrence (2)* used Lioresal® alone,

---

* Note: References for this chapter may be found on page 173.

and with Tegretol. They achieved marked pain relief among patients previously resistant to Tegretol alone. Long term follow-up of those patients indicates continued pain relief for 6 months to four years. They do not mention the dose of Lioresal in the brief article. MSers should plan to find the best dose of Lioresal for tic in a similar manner to that described in Chapter 4.

If Tegretol, or Tegretol and Lioresal, are inadequate to control tic pain, neurosurgeons can eradicate it through surgery, through injection of the trigeminal ganglion or through radiofrequency lesion of the ganglion. No one need suffer the pains of tic douloureux.

Partial Lesions of Sensory Pathways

Plaques in the sensory system often cause complaints like "numbness from here on down." (See Page 308.) But MSers may also develop "nasty irritable sensory change from here on down," or "nasty burning irritable sensory change in just this region." The distribution of these complaints suggests partial lesions of the lateral spinothalamic tract or the entry zone to the dorsal root of an individual segment of the spinal cord. (See Fig. 17-2, page 307.) Neurological examination may reveal mild diminution of pinprick perception in the painful area, but when the pin is finally felt, it is sharper than normal and more disagreeable.

Usually the discomfort is minor and unimportant. Occasionally there is severe pain that requires attention. If you develop nasty, irritating, burning sensory loss that *really* bothers you, Dilantin may make it better. Tegretol will stop it. Try aspirin and related minor pain medications first. Try Dilantin® (See page 171.) to see whether it will interrupt the pain. If these measures prove inadequate, use Tegretol if your discomfort warrants the risk of other side effects. Remember the expense and read about the potential hazards of Tegretol. Decrease the dose periodically, and if pain does not return, stop the medication.

Painful Tonic Seizures

Painful tonic seizures are uncommon among MSers and do not now occur among patients with other illnesses. They were first described by Matthews in 1958 (4) and have had limited recognition since then. The description by Matthews, paraphrased here, is characteristic of these attacks.

"—When putting her left foot to the ground on getting out of bed one morning, she felt a 'peculiar, horrid sensation' in the foot, rapidly spreading up the leg and then involving the left arm. The arm and leg became stiff and she had to sit down. The attack passed off in about 30 seconds. During the next two weeks she experienced similar attacks with great frequency, often having three in 15 minutes and over 30 in a day.

"The attacks began in the left foot and followed a stereotyped pattern, the ankle being turned in and the foot and toes being curled under. The arm was somewhat bent at the elbow and fully bent downward at the wrist and knuckles. The fingers themselves were forcibly straightened. The limbs were held stiffly in this position and she experienced severe pain in the hand and foot.

"Voluntary movement was possible at the

hip and shoulder but not in the hand and foot. There was only stiffness, never any jerking.

"On one occasion she was able to observe herself in a mirror and noticed that her face was drawn up on the left side. She could speak during the attacks but would have to sit down until the attack passed off in about a minute.

... The attacks would occur in bed and sometimes wakened her from sleep, particularly if she turned to lie on her left side.

"Consciousness was neither lost nor disturbed and the attacks were not followed by headache or weakness of the affected limbs. Her doctor prescribed phenobarbital 30 mg. three times a day with immediate cessation of symptoms. On leaving off the tablets for one day soon after starting them, the attacks returned in full force but were immediately controlled again."

Matthews described three other patients with similar attacks. In all four cases the attacks were strictly limited to one side of the body. In three of the four patients the seizures were painful. In all cases, consciousness remained completely normal. Treatment was offered in only two cases because in the other two, the attacks had stopped. One responded well to phenobarbital, the other to Dilantin. Current management includes Tegretol if Dilantin and phenobarbital are ineffective.

Tonic seizures usually stop after a period of time. Plan to stop treatment after several weeks to test whether it is still needed. Start treatment again if spasms return, and wait another few weeks. Eventually you will be able to stop treatment. If the attacks return, resume medication.

These attacks usually occur in MSers with serious disability, although they were the first symptom of MS in one of the patients Matthews reported and in another case described several years later by Joynt and Green (3).

An article by Watson and Chiu suggests that the source of these attacks is a single plaque in the motor system of the brain (5) but this has not been established with certainty. In current practice, tonic seizures are characteristic only of MSers, but very uncommon even among them. This suggests that their occurrence might depend on a special *combination* of lesions in the brain, brainstem and perhaps the cerebellum.

Warning About Use of Tegretol

Tegretol is a potent anticonvulsant which often stops epileptic seizures uncontrolled by other medications. Despite its excellence as an anticonvulsant it is not usually the first medication given to adults. It is expensive and may have serious side effects. The most serious complication, although rare, is death from aplastic anemia.

We use Tegretol to relieve the devastating suffering caused by uncontrolled seizures, betting against the slim chance of aplastic anemia. Throughout this volume we stress the problem of risk *vs.* benefit. There are times in the course of MS when Tegretol becomes a reasonable response to pain. It should be used in those instances for its positive result, while guarding as well as possible against disastrous side effects. Read this section with consideration and forethought, not fear and anxiety.

Aplastic Anemia from Tegretol is
Usually Preventable

Aplastic anemia usually occurs without known cause. The bone marrow stops producing white blood cells, red blood cells and platelets. In this case, a previously healthy person complains to the doctor of fever, sore throat, weakness, fatigue, easy bruising or unusual bleeding. The blood tests disclose far advanced aplastic anemia. Sometimes treatment is effective. Often it is not, and the person dies.

For decades, millions of people have used Tegretol. Aplastic anemia is an extraordinarily rare complication. With early recognition of bone marrow damage, Tegretol can be stopped immediately. This is usually followed by prompt and complete recovery.

Regular Blood Tests Provide Safety

Guard against aplastic anemia caused by Tegretol. Before you take your first tablet, be sure your blood is normal. Then have regular cbc (complete blood count) and platelet counts for as long as you use the medication.

How often should you have a cbc and platelet count? No one can tell for certain. At the beginning, it seems wise to recommend blood tests about every week or two. If, after several months, there is no evidence of bone marrow suppression, testing may be decreased to once a month. If you need Tegretol continuously, cbc and platelet counts may be done four to six times a year for as long as you use Tegretol.

You can manage this issue yourself. If you develop Tegretol-responsive pain and decide to use the medication, plan with your doctor a schedule for regular trips to the laboratory. The day after each test, call the doctor's office to be certain the result was normal. If you assume responsibility in this manner your doctor will be more comfortable with your use of Tegretol, and you can be confident that you are taking charge of *yourself.*

Mild Side-Effects are Common at First

The first doses of Tegretol may cause blurred vision, double vision, vomiting and even staggering. If you start too fast, these side effects can lay you low for days at a time. Such side effects cause no permanent consequence, just temporary discomfort. They are unrelated to aplastic anemia, and are not an MS exacerbation. They merely indicate that your nervous system is unused to the medication. Do you remember your first glass of wine and the sleepiness and unsteadiness it produced? Tegretol acts much the same. As your brain adjusted to alcohol, it will adjust to Tegretol in a week or two. Start again with a smaller dose. Some people must begin with a dose of only 50- to 100 mg. in order to arrive comfortably at an effective dosage regimen.

Severe Side-Effects are Uncommon

Some people can never use Tegretol. Indeed, two of our editors used Tegretol unsuccessfully, one for painful tonic seizures, and the other for pain from a partial sensory lesion. The dose that stopped the man's tonic seizures produced a worse mental disorder. The dose that controlled the woman's pain made her so weak and sick, she preferred the pain! Judge the value of Tegretol against its side effects. If it works well with few side effects, it is worth using. If the benefit is small or the side effects severe, stop it and consider one of these substitutes.

Clifford and Trotter (1) report marked relief of pain through use of tricyclic antidepressant medications like Elavil®. Their description of the different pains differs from ours. Their patients were relieved of many different kinds of MS pain. They used 50–100 mg. per day, which is lower than the recommended dose for treatment of depression.

I have mentioned Dilantin® in other parts of this section. Like Tegretol, Dilantin is an anticonvulsant that can stop some of the MS pains discussed here. It is less effective than Tegretol in controlling these pains, but it is also less toxic. If you have dorsal root entry zone pain, start with Dilantin. The standard dose is 300 mg. each evening. If you have no relief, increase the dose to 400 or even 500 mg. per day. However, at these dosage levels, Dilantin may cause blurred vision, double vision or staggering. If you get pain relief without side effects, Dilantin is your best choice. If you have severe pain that is not relieved by Dilantin, or if you must accept side effects to control it, switch to Tegretol.

There is a great deal of information about Tegretol and Dilantin, which suggests that these medications can damage the developing fetus. Pregnant women should avoid Tegretol, Dilantin and other medications if possible, during at least the first four months of pregnancy.

Dosage Schedules Depend on Side-Effects and Response of Pain to Treatment

If you decide to use Tegretol, begin slowly. One-half tablet (100 mg.) is a proper first dose. If there are no side effects from that dose, take another half tablet after eight to 12 hours. If you still feel fine, increase the dose next day to one-half tablet three times a day. Then increase the dose as rapidly as your side effects allow, until your pain stops. Most people have arrived at an effective dose within a week or 10 days. Tegretol has a biological half-life of eight to 15 hours (See page 87), so most people need three doses in 24 hours.

MS pains usually respond to low doses of Tegretol. People with serious seizure disorder often use 2000 mg. per day. MSers often find relief from pain after the first half-tablet, and at doses of 1000 mg. per day or less.

Unlike seizure disorder, which is a chronic condition, MS pains that respond to Tegretol often last only weeks or months. Therefore, MSers can use Tegretol briefly, then stop temporarily or decrease the dose by 100 mg. per day (one-half tablet) to see if they still need it. If pain does not return after a week, decrease the dose again. Keep yourself on the smallest dose that controls your pain. Eventually, most MSers can discontinue Tegretol and other pain pills until the next attack of pain.

What About Acupuncture? TENS Units? Spinal Cord Implants? All the Other Remedies I Hear About?

People in pain are fair game. Legitimate practitioners try their best to help, but beware of the quacks! If someone recommends special treatment for your pain, investigate, and evaluate the treatment if you can. Try a TENS unit at home before buying it. Decide whether you believe that a pin in your ear lobe will change your nervous system. Read Chapter 20 and evaluate the practitioner who offers treatment. Then, if you want it, and if treatment seems to be safe, spend your money and see if it works.

Remember also, that MSers have all the pains of normal people, plus the pains of MS. As you age, your joints, like mine, will ache. You may have headache, menstrual cramps and stomach pains. Treat pain with respect, not panic. If your pain seems serious, consult your doctor.

REFERENCES:

1) Clifford, D. B.; Trotter, J. L.: Pain in Multiple Sclerosis. *Arch. Neurol.* Vol. 41, Pages 1270-1272, 1984.

2) Fromm, G. H.; Terrence, C. F.: Baclofen in the Treatment of Trigeminal Neuralgia: Double-blind Study and Long Term Follow-up. *Ann. Neurol.* Vol. 14, Page 111, 1983

3) Joynt, R. J.; Green, D.: Tonic Seizures as a Manifestation of Multiple Sclerosis. *Arch. Neurol.* Vol. 6, Pages 293-299, 1962.

4) Matthews, W. B.: Tonic Seizures in Disseminated Sclerosis. *Brain.* Vol. 81, Pages 193-206, 1958.

5) Watson, C. P.; Chiu, M.: Painful Tonic Seizures in Multiple Sclerosis: Localization of a Lesion. *Le Journal Canadien des Sciences Neurologiques.* Vol. 6, Pages 359-361, 1979.

Chapter 9
Management of Exhaustion
By John K. Wolf

Many MSers suffer from unexplained exhaustion before the appearance of any specific symptom of MS. One woman had suffered exclusively from exhaustion for many years. She came for one more consultation after developing trouble walking. She was convinced she had MS. Her husband and her doctors were equally convinced that her problems were psychological, not physical.

All previous laboratory examinations had been normal, including several examinations of the spinal fluid and several CT scans. Even the visual evoked response examination (See page 343.) remained normal when she and I met. Only the neurological examination seemed to have changed. Previous physicians had found abnormal reflexes, but now in addition, Babinski's sign (See page 314.) was, for the first time, present.

She looked fine. She functioned normally except for her fatigue. Her gait was normal when she walked into the office. Why was she tired?

An MRI (See page 335 and Figs. 18-7, 18-8, page 339, 340.) finally and unequivocally demonstrated the presence of a large number of discrete lesions in the white matter of the brain. This study, plus the history and the changes in physical examinations, documented the presence of MS. She was fortunate. She had no paralysis, tremor or sensory loss as so many other MSers do. There was just enough disruption of brain activity to produce exhaustion. Every thought, every association, every action required more effort because damaged portions of the brain could not maintain a smooth chain of command.

I picture such a brain as a series of detours. Neural messages must travel around damaged portions of the brain, just as highway traffic must detour around construction projects. Both use unimproved byways to reach their destination. Any automobile traveler knows the fatigue of such a trip and remembers the relief of smooth tar under the tires again. Imagine spending an entire trip on such roads. Imagine spending an entire life with such detoured neural traffic. Imagine the agony of exhaustion when no definite symptom proclaims MS the cause!

Exhaustion may be a measure of the amount of damage to association pathways in the brain. These pathways facilitate transfer of information from one brain region to another. We have no direct way of measuring damage to these pathways. The neurological examination offers only a gross assessment of the few pathways described in Chapter 17.

Some MSers suffer no exhaustion despite significant paralysis and incoordination. In such people MS plaques may be confined to pathways that transmit specific movement or feeling. Maybe absence of exhaustion in these people means there is little involvement of association pathways in the brain.

For such exhaustion there is no specific treatment, so

MSers must learn to live with it. But spasticity, depression, incoordination, tremor and imbalance *do* respond. As you read this chapter try to discover whether your fatigue may result in part from one of these treatable causes. If so, get treatment and learn to manage better.

TREATABLE CAUSES OF EXHAUSTION

Spasticity

Look again at Chapter 4. Have you done everything you can to reduce spasticity? Spastic muscles work against each other because they receive inaccurate information from the spinal cord. As a leg is thrown forward in walking, spastic muscles on each side of knee and hip joints contract simultaneously instead of waiting their turn as normal muscles do. The spastic leg is pulled in both directions at once. Muscles ache. Walking is slowed. Fatigue becomes exhaustion.

Because spasticity causes loss of power, it requires more effort just to stand up. Muscle strengthening exercises help to improve muscle power even though the exercise itself causes fatigue. It is important to keep your muscles toned up to their best level of function. The energy you spend on exercise is well spent, not wasted. Editor, Diane Tarbell, commented:

"Although I have very mild MS, I found at times when I was not getting enough exercise, I was more fatigued. I would encourage MSers in *all* stages to use their bodies in some sort of regular exercise program. The less severely disabled may benefit even more than more severely disabled folks, in that they are doing something positive, and are mastering and being in control."

176

If muscle strengthening exercises are not enough, aids to mobility can keep you active: Wheelchair, ankle brace, Canadian crutch, walker. Buy them early for use in times of heavy physical activity. Then they will become old friends and trusted allies against future loss of mobility. If you could use aids to ambulation occasionally now, buy them now. Function more efficiently now, and keep yourself mobile despite advancing disability. Now and then, use a wheelchair. Save your energy for activities that interest and please you.

Depression

Exhaustion is a major symptom of depression. If you are weepy and sleepless, if outbursts of anger express depression, and if depression causes fatigue, help is available. Read Chapter 7, to see whether it describes your situation. If it does, get treatment *pronto* and begin to feel human again.

Tremor, Incoordination and Imbalance

The tremor and incoordination of cerebellar disease force muscles of trunk and limbs into a zig-zag course. How much farther than it should, does your body move during a day as you dress, work, eat and play? Each zig and every zag adds to your exhaustion.

Gadgets Counteract Tremor

An electric toothbrush allows MSers to brush their own teeth unassisted despite considerable tremor. Sometimes, wrist weights, held on by Velcro® straps, can dampen tremor if there is little loss of muscle power. One- or two pound weights are usually all people can tolerate. Your occupational therapist has catalogs of ideas about aids to arm and hand mobility. If you have useful ideas for control of arm and hand tremor, please write to us!

Use of Isoniazid for Tremor

Shortly before our first edition of *Mastering Multiple Sclerosis* went to press, an article by Sabra et al. described the use of isoniazid in the treatment of MS tremor (1)*. Our manuscript went to the publisher before we had much experience with its use. Sabra et al. specified one kind of tremor as more responsive than another, but the description was difficult to understand. I now have more experience and can assure MSers that tremor diminishes without serious side effects in some people.

Some MSers appear normal when they sit in a chair or lie quietly in bed. The voluntary movement of feeding themselves or combing their hair, causes tremor that may become extremely severe. When they stop, tremor subsides. In my experience, this kind of tremor has *not* responded to isoniazid.

Other MSers shake during all their waking hours; lying, sitting, working, resting. This tremor does respond to isoniazid. If your tremor is severe and continuous, read on. You may get help. If your constant tremor is mild, or if you have tremor only on voluntary movement, but want to try anyway, read on cautiously. Isoniazid is not always easy to use, and can cause serious side effects.

---

* Note: The reference for this chapter may be found on page 185.

Warnings About Use of Isoniazid

The major dangerous side effect of isoniazid is hepatitis (liver damage). Below the age of 30, the risk of hepatitis is about 0.3%. It rises to 2.3% over the age of 50. The development of hepatitis is not necessarily serious. After isoniazid is stopped, liver function usually returns to normal. Nevertheless, fatal isoniazid hepatitis has been reported. Isoniazid should not be used for trivial tremor, and should be stopped instantly if symptoms of liver damage appear. If you develop gray or yellow bowel movements or frank jaundice, stop isoniazid and call your doctor. If some other symptom suggests liver damage to you while you take isoniazid, call your doctor to check on it.

Use of alcohol during treatment with isoniazid may increase the risk of hepatitis. Do not use alcohol while taking isoniazid.

Because of the danger of hepatitis, have liver function studies done on a blood sample before taking the first dose of isoniazid. If there is evidence of pre-existing liver disease, do not use this medication. Once you start treatment, have liver function studies performed regularly: frequently at first, perhaps every week or two, and then less frequently as you reach your effective dose and gain confidence that your liver will not be damaged.

In Chapter 8 we stressed the importance of taking charge of your own repeated blood studies. (See page 169–170.) The same suggestion applies here. Take charge. Get laboratory slips from your doctor. Discuss together the schedule of liver function studies that will make you both comfortable. See to it that you get to the laboratory to have the studies performed. Then call the office next day to be certain of the result.

Because there is no definite limit to the risk of hepatitis, no one can tell precisely how often nor how long to continue liver function studies. Most hepatitis develops early in the course of treatment, sometimes because of pre-existing liver disease. This is why it is so important to monitor liver function frequently as you begin, then less frequently once you have found your safe dose.

The major symptoms of hepatitis include loss of appetite, nausea, vomiting and jaundice. Bowel movements may lose their normal brown color and become yellow or gray. Bile pigments excreted in the urine turn it dark brown. Should these symptoms appear, stop isoniazid *immediately* and call your doctor.

There is no accurate information about the effects of isoniazid on the developing fetus. Pregnant women should avoid isoniazid, and other medications if possible, for at least the first four months of pregnancy.

Minor Side Effects of Isoniazid

The most common side effect of isoniazid is sleepiness. This may become so severe that the person cannot be wakened. This is not a serious side effect. If isoniazid is stopped, the person wakes again. Some people have become sleepy on as little as 600 mg. per day. There is some tolerance to this side effect, so an MSer who becomes sleepy at a given dose, may later be able to take that dose without trouble.

I treated one woman whose tremor disappeared when she started isoniazid, but she could not stay awake. We found an effective dose for her, but continued to have intermittent trouble, because the effective and the toxic doses were so similar. After she had taken isoniazid for more than a year, I had a series of telephone calls from husband and visiting nurse. She had again gone to sleep and could not be wakened—except to take her pills! We stopped the isoniazid, and two days later she was back to normal.

I mention the two days because isoniazid has a long biological half-life. (See page 87.) Toxic side effects like sleepiness last for several days after isoniazid is stopped. Beneficial effects of the medication do not appear for a week or more after the proper dose has been reached. This is not strictly a side-effect. It is one of the biological characteristics you must keep in mind as you plan treatment strategy.

Pyridoxine Prevents Neuropathy

When isoniazid is used as an antituberculous medication, pyridoxine (vitamin B6) is given at the same time to prevent damage to peripheral nerves. MSers should also use pyridoxine while they take isoniazid. The dose is 50 mg. per day, regardless of the isoniazid dose.

Treatment Strategy with Isoniazid

After all these warnings, you may decide not to take isoniazid. Do not make that mistake. If you have serious continuous tremor, isoniazid can be important to your well-being. If you have mild tremor, or no tremor unless you are eating or doing some other active movement, avoid isoniazid.

If you decide to use isoniazid, remember its long biological half-life. Take your dose only once in 24 hours, not twice or three times a day. Plan to change the dose not more frequently than once every 10 days.

Begin at 300 mg. each bedtime. Chances are this dose will do nothing for you. Ten to 14 days later, increase the dose to 600 mg. a day. Ten days after that, begin to observe the effect on tremor. If there is no change, no sleepiness and no signs of liver damage, then go on to 900, 1200, and 1500 mg. per day, increasing the dose at 10–14 day intervals.

If there is no change in your tremor after 10–14 days on 1500 mg. per day, you will probably get no benefit from isoniazid. If there is some change, consider going to higher doses. But remember, higher doses probably carry an increased risk of hepatitis. Do not continue to take any medication, at any dose, if it fails to produce the desired effect. If you do, you waste your money and increase your risk of side effects.

Since sleepiness may make it impossible for the MSer to manage isoniazid, family members must help with the dosage schedule. If your MSer goes to sleep and can't wake up for meals, stop isoniazid. Once your MSer is back to normal, start again if it has been useful, but at a lower dose.

You cannot get isoniazid without a doctor's prescription, so consider your situation first. Go to the library and read Sabra et al. about use of isoniazid for MS tremor. Bring the information to your doctor and discuss it together. Have liver function studies performed. Plan to increase your dose in a considered and watchful manner. Arrange for family members or frequent observers to watch for sleepiness. If you approach isoniazid and all other treatments with this kind of care, you will have the best chance of success and the fewest side effects.

Imbalance

Spasticity is only one cause of imbalance. Other causes include direct involvement of the cerebellum and its connections (See page 315.), or interruption of conscious and unconscious sensory pathways from muscles, joints and skin. (See page 308.) With no medication to correct imbalance from these other causes, and only marginal benefit from physical therapy, a set of Canadian crutches (See page 16.) can greatly improve your gait and prevent falls.

Sometimes, when MSers fall because of a weak ankle, they mistakenly think imbalance was the cause. Check peroneus and anterior tibial muscle strength. Analyze the reasons for any fall. Were you truly unbalanced, or did the ankle give way? If ankle weakness is the cause of gait disturbance and fatigue, get the ankle splint described on page 20.

Excessive Daily Activities Increase Fatigue

What have you done to conserve your precious energy? Do you continue to try to do things as you always have? Do you believe you should be as productive as you were before you had MS?

Physically healthy people plan their day's work to fit the time and energy available. As they age, they match their daily activities to their lessened energy. MSers must also plan their time and activities to fit available energy reserves.

Are you a night owl who must rise early to get to work? Arrange your bladder management to provide more uninterrupted hours of sleep (Chapter 5). Are you wakeful nights? Can you change your work schedule to allow you to sleep later in the morning and bring work home to do in bed? Can you cut your full-time job to part-time?

More people work at home now, than ever before. This volume was written on a home computer. It has changed my life. Computers have become a major asset for many partially disabled people. If you have the right job, you might modify it to allow you to use a computer at home instead of fighting morning and evening traffic.

Do everything you can to adjust your work to your energy level. Forget goals that require you to "pass for healthy." Forget the artificial requirement to have the same "normal" day you would have had without MS. Establish your priorities carefully. Then pursue important activities unswervingly and reject those that are less important or burdensome. Make changes in your life deliberately. Treat every treatable cause of exhaustion. Be exhausted constructively.

Barbara Shetron's words remain important:

> "All in all, the problems of everyday living are undeniably exhausting. But aren't there good and bad types of exhaustion? Isn't it better to be exhausted from activity than from resting?
>
> "As you know, I have become a great advocate of physical therapy. But if I am going to do arm stretching exercises, I much prefer to do them by washing windows or sweeping floors. Useful activities make me feel better about myself, help keep my body functions intact, and I sure do sleep at night in spite of continuous pain. Does this not work *for* rather than *against* the MSer?"

MS will change your life. No amount of reading and thinking can change the accumulation of plaques in your brain and spinal cord. But changes in life-style can be made with forethought. Think ahead and decide which activities are least important to you and abandon them one at a time. Do not allow disability to rob you of important joys.

RETIREMENT IS NOT ALWAYS THE BEST ANSWER

Do what you can to avoid early retirement. Although retirement looks sweet through the blur of fatiguing days, it is often bitter once the pressure to achieve is removed. Early retirement is almost always permanent. It is lonely to be home. Many people are dissatisfied with early retirement, just as my editor-teacher-friend is with hers. (See page 7.)

The demands of daily work weigh heavily on everyone, healthy or sick. Most employers will try to help you adjust your work schedule so you can continue to be productive despite significant disability. If your job, your employer and your energy can be coordinated, keep working. Then, when you *can't* work any more, find constructive things to do with your time. Volunteer at a local hospital or disabled activist agency. Form a discussion group with other interested people. Read. Visit other MSers who are less fortunate than you are. Keep as busy as your body will allow!

REFERENCES:

1) Sabra, A. F.; Hallet, M.; Sudarsky, L.; Mullally, W.: Treatment of Action Tremor in Multiple Sclerosis with Isoniazid. *Neurology (N. Y.)* Vol. 32, Pages 912–914, 1982.

Chapter 10

Treatment of Acute Exacerbations
By John K. Wolf

I'll outline the course of a typical mild exacerbation that occurred to one of my MSer-friends. The attack had begun six weeks prior to her call. She had had symptoms of left optic neuritis for two weeks. Colors appeared bleached and vision was decreased so she could not read with that eye. As the attack of optic neuritis ran its course, she developed numbness that began in the right thumb and spread through the right arm. Then the entire right side of the body and the right leg went numb. A few days later, numbness spread further to include both sides of the body. She dragged her right leg when she walked. Bowels and bladder functioned well.

She phoned for treatment because for several days she had had double vision and could not drive to work. We would not have treated her for the other symptoms because, frightening as they sound in print, they had not been severe enough to cause significant disability.

Exacerbations are not the same as "bad days," which are major but brief depletions of available energy, unaccompanied by specific neurological symptoms. Exacerbations last for days occasionally, but usually for weeks. During especially troublesome exacerbations, symptoms may follow each other in succession for several months, some symptoms fading while others develop.

The remission that follows is part of the definition of an exacerbation. MSers in the midst of a prolonged attack often wonder: "Will it go away this time as it has in the past?" There is no effective reassurance during a long complicated attack that has tried the patience of MSer, family, doctor and everyone else. Even so, MSers who have experienced previous exacerbations followed by remission, can take heart from those memories. Chances are this one will eventually go away too.

There is also reassurance in the literature. Examine Torben Fog's work in Chapter 19, on the prognosis of MS (page 346). Fog showed that exacerbations are not the cause of MS progression. Examine the Veteran's Administration Study, (page 349) which confirms Fog's conclusions. In the V.A. Study, the frequency, severity and even the specific symptoms of exacerbations did not indicate how severe the illness would be fifteen years later. Read Kurtzke's study of the outcome of individual symptoms of MS (page 351). Symptoms that have been present only briefly usually remit. According to Kurtzke, symptoms present for two years or longer are permanent. But one of our editors commented strongly that his own early disturbance of gait had continued much longer than two years, and had improved dramatically after that time.

Meanwhile, plan to manage this and future exacerbations. As yet, there is no miracle cure that eradicates exacerbations or MS progression, but you can sometimes shorten a bad attack with medication. ACTH and steroid hormones are still the most useful tools in the management of acute exacerbations.

ADRENOCORTICOTROPIC HORMONE (ACTH)

The pituitary gland at the base of the brain manufactures adrenocorticotropic hormone (ACTH). Chemically related to proteins, ACTH is one of several pituitary hormones that govern the function of glands throughout the body. The chief known function of ACTH is to stimulate the adrenal glands to produce steroid hormones. No one knows whether the effect of injected ACTH on MS exacerbations results from its adrenal stimulation or from some other, still unknown action.

The literature on use of ACTH in treating MS is enormous and conflicting. Early reports suggested that ACTH improved the symptoms of MS. Some even suggested it would stop the disease. Later reports have confirmed and denied these results many times. Conflict in the literature means that a treatment is no miracle. The effectiveness of penicillin, for instance, was *never* questioned.

The Cooperative Study. Use of ACTH-Gel in MS Exacerbation

In an attempt to settle the controversy, members of the Schumacher Committee (See page 326.) developed plans for a cooperative clinical trial of ACTH-gel *vs.* placebo in the treatment of acute exacerbations. This trial was organized and performed in 10 major neurological centers. The final result was published in May 1970 (1).*

---

* Note: The reference for this chapter may be found on page 201.

ACTH is available in two forms, a slowly absorbed preparation in a gelatin base (ACTH-gel) for intramuscular (I.M.) injection, and an aqueous form for intravenous (I.V.) use. The Cooperative Study protocol specified use of ACTH-gel in large doses. The purpose was to identify any effect of the treatment that might have been missed by a smaller, inadequate dose.

Before MSers were admitted to the study, they were carefully screened to be certain: 1) that they really had MS, and 2) that they were in the midst of an acute exacerbation. If they met both criteria, they learned about the study. If they wished to participate, they were placed randomly either in a control or a treatment group. There were one hundred and three patients in the treatment group, 94 in the control group. Careful analysis of many factors showed that the two groups were quite similar before treatment.

The treatment group received a two-week course of I.M. ACTH-gel injections. As a direct consequence of the large dose chosen for the study, 44% of the treatment group developed side effects, none of them serious. Thirty-one percent developed acne (pimples). Seven percent developed the puffy face that is characteristic of steroid or ACTH use. Seven percent noted increased hair growth on face, limbs or body. Weight gain or obvious ankle edema occurred in six percent. All these side effects disappeared after ACTH injections were stopped.

Did none of the patients complain of insomnia or depression? In Syracuse, insomnia is the most troublesome side effect of ACTH. Psychological depression was reported in only one patient. In Syracuse, many MSers become at least mildly depressed when they stop ACTH or prednisone. Perhaps the excitement of joining the study prevented significant depression. Maybe the researchers considered insomnia too insignificant to report.

Results of the Cooperative Study

Treatment and control groups were examined carefully at the beginning of the study, and then weekly for the next four weeks. The treatment group was unequivocally in better condition than the placebo group, but the result was statistical, not dramatic. As a group, those who received ACTH were improved. In the individual case the difference was so slight that the researchers could not clearly distinguish treatment from control patients.

Spasticity and gait improved more than any other symptom. The statistical difference was greatest during the early weeks of the study. *By week four, there was no difference at all*. Thus the Cooperative Study provides no support for the long term use of ACTH in the management of MS.

69% of *Untreated* Exacerbations Improved

The Cooperative Study again confirmed the transience of MS exacerbations. Sixty-nine percent of *placebo-treated* patients improved during the four weeks of observation. Keep this important figure in mind when you evaluate reports of some new treatment, or investigate claims by someone who wants your money. Ask for evidence of the effectiveness of their new treatment, and (if you believe they collected information) compare their figures with the known history of an acute exacerbation: 69% of patients improved in four weeks *with no treatment at all*. This does not mean that 69% had returned to baseline in four weeks. They had not, but they were at least starting on the road to remission.

Use of ACTH-Gel in Treatment of Exacerbations

The Cooperative Study provides evidence that ACTH-gel has a limited value in treatment of acute exacerbations. Serious side effects are uncommon if the course of treatment is brief. The chief result of ACTH was a shortened duration and perhaps a lessened severity of the attack.

With these ideas in mind, what sort of attack should be treated? As always, treatment should be better than the disease, so potential side effects must be balanced against potential benefit. A very mild exacerbation that causes no disability should not be treated. In the face of trivial complaints, any side effect would be worse than the symptom. On the other hand, it would be worth your while to be sleepless for a week, in return for a speedy return of power in the legs. A few pimples might be a small price to pay for regained bladder control or improved balance.

Think carefully with your doctor about any exacerbation and its symptoms. During previous courses of ACTH-gel injections, have your symptoms disappeared promptly without troublesome side effects? If an exacerbation causes significant disability, it might be worth your while to treat it. But if you have had several courses of ACTH-gel without improvement, or if you have had severe insomnia, acne, puffy face or other side effect from the medication, avoid the side effects this time and allow the exacerbation to run its course.

Treatment of an exacerbation does not change the long term course of your MS. If you do not treat exacerbations, your progress over the next ten years will be unchanged. The only possible benefit is improvement during the next few weeks. If you decide not to treat, you need not feel you have reached the end of the earth. In the most carefully controlled study, ACTH had only a borderline beneficial effect that became negligible at the fourth week of study.

Suggested Treatment Regimen

Most physicians use smaller doses than those used in the Cooperative Study. Many use smaller doses than the regimen I recommend to my patients. There is no right or wrong dose of ACTH-gel.

I recommend 80 units of ACTH-gel the first day, followed by 40 units a day for about 10 days. The duration of a course of ACTH-gel depends on the response. MSers who improve dramatically in the first three days can stop before the first week is finished. Some MSers receive no benefit after the full 10 days of injections, so we stop at that time to prevent side effects. In still other cases, improvement begins towards the end of the first week or ten days. In such cases we decide to continue the injections for another five to 10 days to get the best possible result. I never recommend daily ACTH-gel injections for longer than 20 days.

Discontinuing ACTH-Gel Injections

There is no need to taper the dose of ACTH-gel as the course of treatment ends. ACTH does stimulate the adrenals, and this stimulation results in shut-down of ACTH production from the pituitary. But the pituitary gland starts producing ACTH again as soon as the injections are stopped.

Unfortunately, *people*, unlike their pituitary glands, cannot always stop ACTH suddenly. During ACTH treatment, some people receive a tremendous "rush" of energy and well-being, and become dependent on ACTH. After ten days of ACTH, some MSers fall into the Depths of Despond as they stop the injections.

This spiritual fall can be prevented. Stop ACTH at the end of your course of treatment. If you become depressed two days later, taper the dose by giving 40 units every other day for three doses (six days), 20 units every other day for three doses (six days), then stop. Some people still have trouble at that level, and taper their dose to 20 units every three days for a few doses before they can finally stop the injections. If this slow withdrawal does not prevent depression, perhaps depression is one of your MS symptoms. Recall your mood before you started ACTH. Read Chapter 7, to see if you are a candidate for Elavil® instead of continuing the ACTH. Talk with your doctor about these issues as they arise!

Technique for Intramuscular Injections

Most MSers can inject ACTH-gel themselves. Get your initial training from your doctor or from a nurse. A professional can easily show you the technique, which seems so difficult and complex in print. A professional can demonstrate injection sites and hold your hand during the first nervous injection. Read on now, but plan to get help when you start.

Keep ACTH-gel refrigerated. The gel solidifies in the cold but liquefies when the vial is held under the hot water tap. Use a 3cc. disposable syringe with a 21 gauge needle. Most people can puncture through to muscle with a one-inch needle. If you are fat, use a 1 1/4 or 1 1/2 inch needle to be certain you inject deep into the muscle, not into the fat under the skin.

Sterilize the rubber top of the bottle with an alcohol swab. Use simple cotton swabs and rubbing alcohol, or the more expensive prepackaged swabs from the pharmacy.

Now think for a moment, because the next step will pull the liquefied ACTH-gel from the bottle. You must replace liquid removed from the bottle with air. If you plan to use one cc. of ACTH-gel, pull slightly more than one cc. of air into your syringe. Then insert the needle into the center of the rubber stopper of the bottle. If you have a long needle, and hold the bottle upside down, the tip may be above the fluid level if you insert the needle all the way, and you cannot remove the medication. So put only the *tip* of the needle into the bottle. Push the air into the bottle and pull out your dose. Hold the syringe needle-end up, and flush any remaining air bubbles into the bottle. You would not be harmed if you injected those bubbles into your muscle, but air bubbles rob you of just that much ACTH. So get rid of them.

The easiest injection sites are the anterior (top) or lateral (outside) surface of the thigh (between hip and knee), immediately available when you sit down. They are a large enough target to hit, even if you have significant visual loss or tremor. There are no vital organs or major blood vessels near the top and outside of the thighs so you cannot hurt yourself. Avoid the medial (inner) side of the thigh. The femoral nerve, artery and vein run there and could be damaged by an injection. Besides, the skin there is more sensitive than on the rest of the thigh, so the shot would hurt more.

Pull air into the syringe. Withdraw your dose from the vial. Swab off the skin where you plan to inject the medicine—and stick the needle in, all the way to the hub.

Once you have the needle in place, pull back slightly on the plunger to be certain the needle tip is not in a blood vessel. Have your instructor show you this important move, because ACTH-gel is not formulated for I.V. use. If blood does come back when you pull back, move to another injection site and carry on. Blood in the syringe has no effect on the medication. Do not waste the dose.

There are many more than ten injection sites on the top and outsides of your two thighs. During a course of ACTH-gel injections, move your injection sites systematically from left to right, and up and down your thighs.

The advantages of self-injection go beyond the obvious saving of time and money spent in the doctor's office or waiting for the visiting nurse. MSers are plagued by many things they cannot do for themselves. By self-injection, you have preserved one more important function. Take the family out to dinner with the money saved, to celebrate your continued independence.

Cautions and Warnings About ACTH-Gel Injection

Many people, especially women, develop unsightly black and blue marks at injection sites. These are of no consequence and will disappear in several months. You can prevent most of these marks by being certain to inject into the muscle, not the fat under the skin. Use a long enough needle. Insert it to the hub and inject deeply.

Infection is almost never a problem. Should an injection site become infected, it would feel hot, appear red, and unless you have sensory loss, it would hurt. If you develop infection in an injection site, call your doctor immediately, or go to the nearest emergency room for care.

All diabetics should use ACTH cautiously, because diabetes often becomes uncontrolled during a course of treatment. MSers with "brittle" (hard to control) diabetes should avoid ACTH in any form unless they are hospitalized. The slight benefit from the injections would easily be outweighed by any diabetic complication.

Always avoid the medial (inner) surface of the thigh when you inject.

There is no accurate information about the effects of ACTH or steroids on the developing fetus. Pregnant women should avoid ACTH, steroids and other medications if possible, for at least the first four months of pregnancy.

Common Side-Effects of ACTH-Gel

Compared to many other medications, ACTH-gel is safe, if used with care. Insomnia is the most annoying side effect. The "rush" from a morning injection continues through the day and into the night, leaving the MSer tossing and turning. Sleeping pills have a valid place in treatment of short-lived insomnia, but even sleeping pills may not put you to sleep during a course of ACTH-gel. Sleeplessness is uncomfortable but not damaging. If you develop severe insomnia, plan to read James Michener's *Centennial*, or *The Source* during your course of treatment, or some other good book, so you can enjoy your wakeful nights.

Ankle swelling is troublesome to MSers with severe weakness of the legs. Ankle swelling may be partially prevented by restricting salt during the course of treatment. If necessary, it may be further reduced with diuretic tablets. If you use diuretic tablets frequently, replace lost potassium by eating bananas and oranges. Commercial potassium supplements are available by prescription. MSers with severe edema probably have some other trouble, and should ask a doctor about it.

Troublesome acne and facial puffiness disappear during the first two or three months after treatment. Increased hair growth is more persistent, but usually not disfiguring.

INTRAVENOUS ACTH

Aqueous ACTH is formulated for intravenous (I.V.) use. Intravenous therapy is an extraordinary measure, reserved for inpatient use. Some MS exacerbations are so severe that hospitalization is indicated. In this situation, use of I.V. ACTH might easily be included as part of the treatment.

In *theory,* an I.V. drip of ACTH that lasts for 12 hours should be more potent than an I.M. shot. No one has studied this question. In theory, the use of 100 units of ACTH in the I.V. should do more of whatever ACTH does than the 40 units in the I.M. injection. No one has studied this question. In theory, therefore, a 10-day course of 100 units aqueous ACTH, given I.V. each day over a 12 hour period, should *really* benefit an MSer who has failed to respond to less aggressive therapy. No one has studied that question, either.

Even so, there are MSers who respond dramatically during a course of I.V. ACTH therapy, who had made no progress during a course of I.M. injections or steroid tablets. (See page 199.) Some MSers enter the hospital for I.V. ACTH in the midst of a devastating exacerbation and leave walking. Comparison to the former course of the exacerbation makes it unlikely that the improvement merely represents the natural course of that exacerbation.

Without controlled studies, we fall back on belief, on hope, and on admittedly inaccurate "clinical experience." I believe I.V. ACTH is more effective than I.M. I hope I am right. When I think the trouble warrants aggressive measures, I recommend it.

Complications and Potential Benefits of I.V. ACTH

An I.V. course of ACTH has complications and warnings similar to those for an I.M. course. Occasionally, hypertension flares up. Occasionally there is potassium depletion. I.V. sites may become inflamed. Veins may thrombose. These complications are easily diagnosed and treated in the hospital setting.

Hospitalization exposes MSers to unique hazards as well as benefits. Popular movies have emphasized the hazards of hospitalization, but the benefits are also important. Hospital professionals may have time to teach skills of self-care. Daily contact with physical and occupational therapists may offer you a better exercise program. Conversations with the hospital social worker may improve your understanding of home and family situations, or may lead to a better program of home care on discharge. If your hospitalization includes these contacts, you will probably return home better equipped to manage. If the symptoms are serious, the benefits of hospitalization usually outweigh the disadvantages.

STEROID HORMONE TABLETS

Prednisone and other steroid hormone tablets may be as effective in the treatment of an exacerbation as either form of ACTH. No one has studied this question. Some MSers report dramatic improvement during a course of steroid therapy. We would need a cooperative controlled study to prove the tablets were the reason for improvement. Such a study would be expensive, and that money can be better spent on other things.

There are two reasons to use steroid hormone tablets instead of ACTH-gel shots or I.V. ACTH. First, squeamish MSers may prefer tablets to injections. Second, we hope the tablets may be as effective as the ACTH, even though a controlled trial has not been done.

The MSer who hates shots may decide to use Prednisone, 40 mg. per day for 10 days to see if there is a change for the better. If there is no change, or if the exacerbation continues to worsen, reconsider. Perhaps the possible benefit of I.M. ACTH-gel, or of hospitalization for I.V. ACTH might outweigh the disadvantages. You can still switch, despite your initial dislike of those options.

Complications of Steroid Treatment

Most complications of steroid treatment are identical to those of ACTH. There are, however, additional complications to steroid therapy. During the course of treatment, the adrenal glands become dormant. If steroid treatment is prolonged, cells in the adrenals may atrophy. You can avoid this unfortunate result by limiting the course of steroid treatment to 10 to 20 days, and by tapering the dose toward the end of treatment. MSers who have had steroid tablets for only 10 days usually do not need to taper the dose, because adrenal atrophy does not occur that fast. If you take the tablets for 20 days, 40 mg. per day, taper to 40 mg. every other morning for three doses (six days), 20 mg. every other morning for three doses (six days), and then stop.

TREATMENT OF STEADILY PROGRESSIVE MS

MSers with steady progression usually respond less well to ACTH or steroids than those treated for an exacerbation. Even so, some MSers with steadily progressive MS may improve significantly from a course of ACTH-gel injections or Prednisone tablets. It is certainly worth a single trial if you have significant disability. Talk to your doctor. Try a course of treatment. Evaluate the result critically. Ignore the rush of well-being the shots or tablets give you. Concentrate on the degree of improvement you received during and after the course of treatment. Is your walking really better? Does the improvement last? If so, perhaps it might be worth your while to take a 10-day course each year. If there is only marginal improvement or none, do not repeat the experiment.

CHRONIC TREATMENT WITH STEROIDS

There is no established indication for prolonged treatment of MS with steroids or ACTH. The long-term side effects of daily treatment are serious and potentially crippling. Additionally, there is no credible evidence that these medications improve the long term course of multiple sclerosis.

Some MSers who are barely able to function in jobs or at home find that once- or twice-weekly injections of 20 to 40 units of ACTH-gel give them just enough of a boost to help them continue cherished activities. There is little danger from twice-weekly injections of ACTH. If they really help to maintain function, perhaps they are justified.

REFERENCE:

1) Rose, A. S., et al.: Cooperative Study in the Evaluation of Therapy in Multiple Sclerosis *vs*. Placebo. Final Report. *Neurology* (Minneap.) Vol. 20 (No. 5 Part 2), 1970.

Chapter 11

Capsules and Pills Cure
All of Your Ills
(Or Do They?)
By John K. Wolf

Most of us in the caring professions want to help people. With this incentive, we investigate complaints to arrive at accurate diagnosis and effective treatment. Diagnosis—treatment. Diagnosis—treatment. It becomes a reflex with us but, like MSers, we sometimes develop *hyper*-reflexia, and that leads to trouble.

Diagnosis and proper treatment of complaints like nervousness, anxiety attacks, anger outbursts, sleeplessness or family fighting, depend upon knowledge of their frequency and severity. MSers have these problems just as other people do, and solve them about as well. But MSers also have ready access to a physician's ear. If an MSer is sleepless, the doctor is a telephone call away, and the office is accessible. A doctor is not so easily available to most people, so they carry on alone unless the trouble is serious.

Confronted with one of these complaints, a hyper-reflexic doctor may simply prescribe. But pills are usually not the best answer and they can cause problems of their own. Consider these two most common complaints: sleeplessness and "nerves."

SLEEPLESSNESS

"I go to bed exhausted, but I can't sleep."

"I fall asleep immediately, but I wake up at two in the morning and lie awake for hours."

"I never sleep."

"Please refill my prescription for sleeping pills."

Most people who complain of insomnia sleep normally. They merely sleep less well than they wish they could and resent it. Most of us wish we could sleep more soundly. As we grow older, our sleep habits become increasingly irritating. It is normal for older people to wake more frequently during the night than they used to. If middle aged and older persons do not know this, they assume they suffer from insomnia. A few people do have truly serious insomnia, but *no one* requires the automatic use of sleeping pills every night.

There is no harm in having sleeping pills on hand for occasional use. If you have a special event and must sleep beforehand, use a pill. If you plan a long airplane ride and want to sleep through it, use a pill. For occasional use, a sleeping pill will be effective, because your body has not grown resistant and responds to the medication.

When sleepers are used every night, the advantages of occasional use are lost. The brain simply adjusts to frequent sedation, sets its excitability level slightly higher, and wakes anyway at the usual hour. Now the wakefulness is worse because the sufferer hoped to sleep, but wakes to worry—about the second or third pill of the night as *well* as everything else!

Sleeping pills are not especially dangerous. They are expensive. Sometimes they leave a morning hangover that lasts till noon or later. They can lead to serious habituation and this *is* a problem. Sleeping pills are Controlled Substances, requiring special prescriptions from the doctor who may ask those embarrassing questions about how you use them. Then there are those secret thoughts about getting prescriptions from more than one source, and going to more than one pharmacy. Abusers waste a lot of time and energy on such considerations. If you do not now abuse medications, don't start.

Kick the Sleeper Habit

If you are a confirmed pill-o-holic who wants to stop, but know you cannot do it without help, ask around. You can get help in drug rehabilitation units in many towns and all cities. Once you are off the pills, tricks suggested in this section can help you stay off. But first, get the help you need.

If you already have the sleeper habit but are not a confirmed pill-o-holic, ask yourself if the pills really help you.

> Have you become their night time slave?
> Will you tolerate slavery?
> For how long?
> Why?
> Maybe instead, you could kick the habit.

Try to do it yourself first. Begin by putting away the sleepers and downers. Then give yourself a fighting chance. Avoid coffee, tea and other caffeinated drinks after 3:00 P.M. Be as active as you can during the day and stay out of bed until you are sleepy. When you finally go to bed, bring with you a book, radio or TV. Read or listen until you become drowsy. You may be awake and listening till far into the night this first time, but be of good cheer, the morning will come on time.

You may not sleep at all that first night, as your surprised nervous system waits for the expected dose. Get up next morning as usual. Work hard again. Avoid an afternoon nap and stay up until you are sleepy. Chances are, tonight you'll be in bed earlier and may sleep a little. If you persevere for a week, you will sleep. Despite that, you will probably remain permanently dissatisfied with your sleep habits.

The end of the first week is a good time to throw away the pills. The temptation to return to them will increase, and become stronger before it finally weakens and gives you peace. It is hard to give up a chemical habit like sleepers, alcohol or cigarettes. But only the first six to eight *years* are the hardest. During that time you will experience a sudden overwhelming need! If the pills are still in the house you may lose your iron ill. So throw them away after the first week and never allow them into your house again.

After a month off the pills, you may find an absolutely airtight reason for taking a sleeper—just this once—because of some important event next day. Don't do it. On those awful nights when you crave a pill, get out of bed. Read. Watch TV. Listen to an all-night talk show. Call in and complain about insomnia and see what response you get on the radio! Work on hobbies. Clean the kitchen. Exercise. Stay up until you are sleepy again, but then get up at the usual time. Go about your usual business during the day so you can sleep that night.

Constantly at first, but now and then for the rest of your life, you will have restless nights when you will crave chemicals. On those nights, you may find yourself mentioning the name of Our Lord and this author in the same sentence. That's OK. I can take it for a night or two and He (She?) is accustomed to it. After six or eight years, your craving will subside and your profanity will diminish, but your susceptibility to the habit will continue.

I know. I am a reformed two-pack-per-day smoker since the spring of 1958. For years after I stopped smoking, I suffered the pangs I describe above. I *still* walk down hospital corridors behind smokers, inhaling what they exhale. Were I to smoke a cigarette now, I could probably not stop there, so I avoid them like the plague.

If you do finally lie back to go to sleep, do not demand instant oblivion. Sleep research discloses that most people spend many minutes falling asleep. You will too, especially on those first, terrible nights without pills. Conscious relaxation is sometimes effective to induce sleep when it will not come spontaneously. Think of your toes and relax them. Wait until you feel them relax before you move on to relax muscles of your calves and your knee joints. Think of the warmth and looseness in those parts and then move on to your thighs. Relax your pelvis. Snuggle it down into the mattress and think of the warmth in your belly and genital region. Relax your whole body, part by part, and feel it settle into the bed. Take 20 minutes. Check frequently to be certain all parts stay relaxed. If you do this, your body will rest even if you have a sleepless night.

A visiting nurse who read this section suggested imagining a moving warm red light shining on the body, warming parts sequentially. The imagination is yours. Think of the things that relax you.

Other Treatable Causes of Insomnia

Sometimes the complaint of insomnia represents treatable depression. Read Chapter 7 to determine whether your sleeplessness is a result of depression. If so, it might be wise to use an antidepressant rather than sleeping pills.

Physical symptoms keep some people awake. Spasticity is especially troublesome to MSers who have not yet found Lioresal®. Re-read Chapter 4 to see whether you might need Lioresal, or if you already do, whether a change in your dosage schedule would provide more peace at night.

Bladder dysfunction wakens people repeatedly. Have you done everything you possibly can to eliminate the need to get up at night to urinate? Read through Chapter 5, to see if you can find tricks to let you sleep.

The need for sex sometimes causes insomnia. In that case, wake your partner and see what can be made of it. Those times are often the most fun! Then both of you can cuddle and go back to sleep again.

If you have no partner, or if your partner is uninterested and you recognize the need, learn to masturbate. You may even discover that you have found the perfect partner. Who else knows your every pleasure? Who knows better where you are sensitive and where you are not? During solitary sex, there is no intrusion on your privacy. Relief of sexual tension is immediately available without the risk of exploitation or rejection. If you are sleepless because of sexual excitement, relieve it and go back to sleep.

There are many other causes of sleepless nights: exciting events of the day, family arguments, money problems and much more. If problems keep you awake, find the solution. If there is no solution, decide how to live with them. Do not lie in bed and fret. Turn on the lamp. Problems shrink in lighted rooms. Get out pen and paper or tape recorder. Make lists of options if that helps you. When you have done what you can, go back to bed, relax and sleep. You will survive.

Sleep Apnea

Very few MSers have sleep apnea. I include this section because sleep apnea is a treatable cause of nighttime trouble and daytime sleepiness. If readers with sleep apnea recognize themselves and get treatment, this section will have done its job.

"Apnea" means cessation of breathing. People with sleep apnea stop breathing repeatedly while they sleep. This usually occurs in a fat person. It is caused by the weight of fat on trachea (breath pipe) and throat. Because of great weight and extra tissue in the area, these passages close completely and obstruct breathing. The major symptom is enormous snoring, interrupted by periodic complete obstruction. Anxious spouses who turn on the light can see the chest heaving against the obstruction. The breathing stops, sometimes for 60 seconds or more, and then resumes with loud heavy snores. This cycle is repeated over and over all night long.

People with obstructive sleep apnea wake repeatedly, but only partially, during the night. In the morning they may remember dreaming that they couldn't breathe.

When awaking at night, they are often groggy with sleep and lack of oxygen. They thrash around and may strike out wildly. Such behavior is not calculated to improve marital bliss in a double bed!

Because sleep is constantly interrupted during the night, sleep apnea sufferers may immediately fall asleep during the day when they sit down. Charles Dickens immortalized sleep apnea without knowing the cause. It has since been called the Pickwick Syndrome.

Obstructive sleep apnea is curable, either through a chronic tracheostomy, which can be opened during the night to prevent obstruction, or through use of certain medications. If you believe you or your spouse has sleep apnea, ask for referral to a medical center with a sleep laboratory. Your neurologist may know where to send you.

"NERVES"

"I'm jumpy as a cat!" (Where did that expression originate? Certainly not from cats I have known.)

"I fly off the handle at the least provocation."

"I am too shy to go out in public."

"Everything is going to pieces. Our son was arrested for speeding and must go to court again. Our daughter's friends play the stereo full blast in the basement and drive us crazy. Last night the bed fell down and crushed the cat. I can't stand any more!"

Most MSers who complain of "nervousness" are

simply normal people, who live in troubled times. Things happen too fast. Too many other people need too much and it is not there to give. MSers call when they think they have reached their limit. Pressures of family, job, money, housing, sex, transportation all add to the already burdensome pressures of disability. Some people get ulcers. Others have headaches. Still others feel nervous.

Medical hyper-reflexia leads to the automatic prescription of major or minor tranquilizers for thousands of patients who might get along better without them. People bring their nervousness with them into the consultation room. Nervous patients leave doctors and nurses shaken and nervous themselves. Other patients end the consultation and leave, but nervous people stay, waiting for help. The urge to prescribe and end the interview is overwhelming.

"Here. Take this. You will feel better
(—And so will I)."

It takes courage and extra time to face a nervous patient who asks for pills, and to turn the conversation to other treatment options. The busy day is already crowded. Doctors do not have extra time for counseling. Some physicians lack knowledge of community resources, so they cannot make excellent referrals to family counseling agencies, social workers, clinical psychologists, psychiatrists. In many communities, there *are* no resources. So we prescribe.

Sometimes we prescribe for the moment, without thinking about the long term complications of the decision. Some of us take the easy way out to shorten the office visits of nervous people, so we can go on to care for other patients we understand better. "Here.

210

Take this." Some of us believe this response is a good one. Sometimes it is.

Like sleeplessness, the complaint of "nerves" may mask treatable depression. If depression is the cause of nervousness, help is immediately available. Read Chapter 7 again and consult your doctor.

Some MSers have severe psychosis or other emotional illness. In this situation, complaints of nervousness are merely the tip of an emotional iceberg. If your complaint of nervousness means that you really cannot function in the family or outside the home because of severe emotional turmoil, you may need prompt psychiatric consultation.

SUMMARY

We all live with pressure. Symptoms occur when pressure exceeds our ability to cope. Usually we find the needed strength and carry on anyway. Pills complicate things. They delay decisions or allow them to be made by a mind dulled with chemicals. If you use chemistry to keep you comfortable, yesterday's problems will not go away. And today's problems have just begun!

Families with MS face special stresses that other families do not have. Even so, most MS families can avoid chemically induced tranquility. Tranquilizers and sleepers dull the pleasures of life as well as the pain. A tranquil person may remember joyful events of the day, but cannot participate fully. Families recognize this and begin to ignore a tranquil person, rather than to encourage full participation. We are bereft of too many joys. Preserve those you can by keeping your brain alive and aware.

Prozac
New Antidepressant

Addendum March, 1989: Since this book was published, a new antidepressant, Prozac (Fluoxetine Hydrochloride), has been released. Prozac is effective, easy to use, and has fewer annoying side effects than Elavil. Depressed MSers who have not responded to best doses of Elavil may improve with Prozac.

Treatment strategies are similar to Elavil, but the regimen is simpler. Start with one 20 mg. capsule each morning and wait two weeks before increasing the dose. Some MSers require 20 mg. morning and noon. Maximum dose is 80 mg./day.

Side effects: Mild nausea may lead to modest weight loss. Diarrhea is occasionally troublesome. Insomnia, nervousness and excitement are usually absent or mild. Dry mouth and sedation that accompany Elavil, disappear on Prozac.

Unlike Elavil, some patients report improved mood within days of starting Prozac, even though its biological half-life is two to three days, and an active breakdown product has an even longer, 7 - 9 day half-life. Because of its long biological half-life, a given dose may not reach full effectiveness for a month or more.

Warning: Prozac is eliminated through the liver. MSers with liver disease should consult carefully with an internist or a psychiatrist before using Prozac. There is no accurate information about the effects of Prozac on the developing fetus. Pregnant women should avoid Prozac, and other medications if possible, during at least the first four months of pregnancy. The manufacturer's package insert is the best source of current prescribing information for Prozac.

Section Three

Management of Interpersonal Relationships

Introduction

Multiple Sclerosis accentuates life's uncertainty. There is no script. Predictions are impossible. Planning is difficult. Chapters in this section address many of the interpersonal issues that confront MSers and their families. It is possible to master relationships with other people, just as it is possible to manage the physical symptoms of MS. But mastery is not control. Through study and practice we *can* cope with the problems, the tasks and the people. Thus we gain control of our own situation, and so live better and contribute more.

Think about your personal relationships and about the way the people around you interact. Learn how you and your family can strengthen your relationships.

Families, not individuals, must face MS. Chapter 12 emphasizes the importance of family in chronic illness. I hope that our broad definition of family will help you to understand how family members and MSers respond to the disease. The Family Life Cycle idea can broaden your outlook on the unique impact of MS on the family. The family grows and changes as a unit. The cycles of family life put MS into a new perspective, as another challenge of the life cycle.

Resources of maturity, memory and time, plus religious faith can continue to be utilized as illness progresses. MSers have written to us that their religious faith has been an important resource. The Rev. Nancy Chaffee contends that religion puts suffering in its proper perspective. Finally, self-esteem is also presented in a family, not individual perspective.

In Chapter 13 we discuss the impact of MS on marriage and intimate relationships. Marriages that work require flexibility for the major role changes often necessary in long term illness. Fighting is presented as a necessary part of intimacy, something to do better, not less. Some marriages work, others will not. If yours does not, you will need to cope with the extra tasks of separation, divorce, and the rebuilding of new relationships.

Parenting in MS families is the topic of Chapter 14. Children will tell us much when we watch and listen carefully. In MS families, the needs of children can be carefully separated from those of the illness. A disabled parent can still parent. Some ideas are presented to decode and respond to the puzzling behavior of children.

Chapter 15, Sexual Enhancement for MSers and Partners, was written by an MS couple who felt that sexual issues were given short shrift in the first edition of this volume. They filled the gap by presenting a frank, joyous discussion for this edition. Bernice Gottschalk and Mike Sarette challenge the reader to seek physical intimacy and pleasure, together *or* alone.

Finally, a chapter on managing the patient-doctor relationship. John suggests that if you understand your doctors, you may be better able to manage your relationship with them. As I read that chapter, I thought: struggling is an inevitable part of managing. Good luck, I say!

Adaptability

Think for a moment about adaptation. Individuals and families adjust in varying ways to chronic illness. One family has great difficulty accepting illness, while another does it with grace.

Early family experiences influence personality development. In a loving and secure environment, a baby learns to trust, and may later be able to reach out to others. Childhood proceeds through other stages of emotional and intellectual development. These determine how we feel about ourselves. Are we masters of our own fate? Do we influence the world around us? Genes, parents, early upbringing, all contribute to our adaptive abilities.

What resources have we for making a big adjustment? The body and personality we were given, a capacity to reason and to make choices about our lives. We can learn to think of ourselves as choosers, not passive drifters. The very process of choosing and knowing that there *are* choices can help us adapt.

Your authors presume that better information, heightened awareness, and objectivity are useful tools for coping with chronic illness. The information presented may expand your own awareness. We hope it will increase the choices available to you for managing important relationships in your life.

Chapter 12
Family Relationships and MS
By Mitzi Wolf

THE MODERN FAMILY

For our purposes, *a family is any collection of people who live together with a commitment to the welfare of all.* It is a place of nurture, and a sanctuary from the outside world. Families civilize us. Families enrich the physical and emotional, as well as the intellectual sides of our personality. We can be tolerated in our family despite our shortcomings, and celebrated there for our gifts. When we are away, we can pretend to be more rational and competent than we really are, but at home we can be real. The main purpose of a family is to provide sanctuary for its members, a safe harbor for people to be at their worst, to pout, or withdraw for a time. Families can offer kindness and understanding for irrational as well as rational behavior. By confronting our foibles and accepting us anyway, families help us to improve personal relationships at home and away

Contemporary life has dramatically changed our ideas of family. The traditional mother, father and 2.3 children is no longer the only unit. Indeed that kind of family may be a minority by the end of this century. Increases in the divorce rate, in single parent and remarried families have led to new family groups. Now, nearly one of every six children in the U.S. is a step-child. Couples live together in increasing numbers. Three generation families (parent-adult-child) often develop around a person with chronic illness. Even staff and residents in nursing home and residential care facilities form family units.

The broad definition of family used in this volume includes all these groups. I hope these chapters challenge you to manage better in your family relationships. As you read, consider the quality of your current family life. By working together, can you improve it?

BEWARE OF STEREOTYPES AND IDEALS

The traditional stereotype of the normal American family is misleading. The ideal family does not exist. The stereotype does—in a child's first reader and magazines, in TV commercials. The smiling, two parent family has a polished, slim, beautiful wife-mother-goddess who can do everything. She solves problems with grace and wisdom, every hair in place. The handsome, successful husband-father-wise man sits at the wheel of his elegant car, always reasonable, with an answer to every question. The 2.3 children are clean. They smile, are never sullen, belligerent or messy. TV simplifies family life with half-hour solutions to all problems. There is a whisper of magic in these TV dramas. As MSer families watch such programs, they are transported to a fantasy world, where nobody has MS, nobody struggles, and nobody makes monthly payments.

Magical television families trap everyone to some extent. They are especially painful to MSer families, who often feel different from others anyway. Unless the stereotype of normal family life is recognized for what it is—a commercial image—it can cause trouble.

Real families, with or without MS, have trouble. We all struggle. We all have problems. Although fantasy is important, it can also mislead us and our children. So beware of stereotypes and the hidden pressures they place on everyone. All relationships require an investment of time and effort.

TAKING STOCK AND TAKING ACTION

Adults need nurture, sanctuary and education as much as babies do. Think how your family nurtures and affirms all members—children and adults. In MSer families, the need for physical care is obvious. But if the couple concentrates too heavily on physical care, the emotional needs of MSer and care giver may be neglected.

How about the teaching function of your family? Does your family teach each member how to live within the family and away? As the years go by, does the whole family continue to learn and relearn about MS?

Sit down with your family and talk about your mutual needs for emotional expression, for growth, for change. Ask yourselves what life is like in your home. How do you treat each other? How much time do you spend arguing, having fun, talking? How do you and your partner communicate with each other? When you disagree, are you more negative or positive? Does your family affirm every member, and how does it do it? Do you tell the others how lovable and capable they are? Or does one member get more criticism and less praise? Do they appreciate you? Who does the chores—one person only? How do you prepare your children to grow up and leave home? How do they learn to work, to share, to be considerate of others? Are they able to establish their own life goals?

As you discuss these questions together, set some family objectives, and some personal goals. Then work on them. If you have trouble talking alone as a family, join a church group, an independent family discussion group, or form an MS discussion group in your community. MS complicates family life. But the quality of life can be improved in all families by taking stock, setting goals, establishing priorities and changing attitudes and behavior. Although these questions are geared toward *group* discussions, one thoughtful family member can improve the quality of family life.

REACTIONS TO DIAGNOSIS: EVERYBODY IS AFFECTED

A crisis complicates everything we do. Initially we become disorganized. Some can grow through a crisis, and emerge better able to cope. Others are overwhelmed and defeated. Common first reactions include denial, feelings of helplessness, shame, fear, and anger. Add this to the ordinary strains of family life, and you have a family in turmoil.

Symptoms develop slowly in MS, so MSer and family can deny its presence. This may be a healthy response. MSers have reported both positive and negative consequences of denial. Sometimes denial kept them going, trying, working at a job, not giving in. Sometimes it continued too long. Children reported parents driving the car when coordination and vision were impaired, still insisting they were capable. Partners of MSers may deny because they desire a well partner. On the other hand, the expectation that the MSer *can* perform well until proven otherwise, can be a big help to the whole family.

What about the fear? One spouse wondered if anyone could ever understand that gigantic fear. The reality is that it will be there. It is normal and necessary, before the next step can be taken. When we are afraid or despairing, we tend to withdraw. When we withdraw, we are less able to help one another. Expect short tempers. Expect feelings to be on the surface. Expect little problems to seem big. Expect each person in the family to feel and transmit fear differently. Children are more concrete and open with fears. Their nightmares may increase. Sleep disturbances and nervous habits are likely to multiply for all family members.

Early reactions are not limited to fear and denial. There is also anger, resentment, frustration and sadness. Guilt complicates the whole scene. "I shouldn't feel this way. After all, I don't even *have* MS!" One 15 year old girl saw that her father was not in control. For the first time in her life, he was afraid, and that frightened *her*. Nobody talked. They kept to themselves. Her father had never expressed emotions. Now he blew up in front of the family. His fear frightened her. She wanted to run away from the problem, but being the oldest, she felt she had to protect the younger children. She did this by *appearing* strong, while actually withdrawing into herself.

Another girl recalled that when she was six, and her father was diagnosed with MS, she wondered if he was angry at *her*! She could not understand his fury. When he threw things, she left the house, to avoid being the object of his wrath. She watched him weep, and hurt for him. At that age, she had no understanding of his illness, nor of his response to it. Children often tell us graphically and concretely about the denial, fear, withdrawal and sadness they have felt.

MANAGING

What can you do about this? First of all, expect it. Expect to be confused and mixed up, to feel afraid, and overwhelmed. Expect to pull inward. Be aware that it will take time to overcome these feelings. Move into your sadness and confusion so you can experience them fully. Expect less of yourself and of others at this time. Parents need to deal with their *own* feelings before they can help their children. The two girls mentioned above remind us that the children are often *left out* in a family crisis. Their emotions are the same as MSers and partners, but they have fewer coping skills.

Sit down together to talk about the diagnosis. You may want a counselor to help with the conversation. Look for a person who understands families and MS. Your minister? Your doctor? A family friend? A professional family counselor? Talk about how people are reacting. Discuss feelings and reactions openly. By admitting their fear, confusion, and sadness in such a conversation, parents can be models for their children. Discussions can help all family members become involved in the diagnosis, and learn how MS will change their lives. This in itself can decrease some of the isolation.

Children may need an outsider to whom they can air their reactions, in addition to family conversations.

How helpful can your doctor be? That depends on the doctor. Many MSers report that doctors are abrupt and do not discuss family issues. Try to understand your physician's despair at having had to diagnose MS.

Realize also that your family doctor is untrained in family counseling. What do you do when your family confronts this new problem? You seek facts. The facts in this book can begin to calm the shock waves. Ask the local MS Society for information. Often relatives can be helpful. Gear discussions with your children to their level of understanding. Ask a sensitive teacher, youth leader, or family member to lead them. One rehabilitation counselor recommends a course in assertiveness training, as a good way to give perspective to the many conflicting emotions (9).*

Family Survival with MS: The Long Haul

The whole family participates in facing MS and planning for the long haul. Both positive and negative issues emerge during this period. Some of these problems have been covered in other chapters. The last approach is to consider all issues from the perspective of the whole family.

THE LIFE CYCLE OF THE FAMILY: The Life Cycle of Multiple Sclerosis

Recently, much has been written about the cycles of life. Eric Erickson talked about the stages of life and the individual challenges that accompany each age (8). More recent writers like Carter and McColdrick, Levinson, and Sheehy, have added other dimensions to the life cycle idea (5, 12, 16).

What is the family life cycle? It is a way of thinking about families and their progress through life. We

---

* Note: References for this chapter may be found on pages 235 and 236.

develop along a continuum in families. There are specific challenges for each life period. For example, a young married couple must learn to relate to both sets of parents. They must readjust when children come, and again when parents get old. If these jobs are clearly understood, couples may diminish the struggles with their parents. Transitions from one stage to another create family pressure. Illness itself is a big transition. It can come at any time in the life cycle, and involves a new set of challenges and problems. What about the MS family? Not only must the members understand the disease, but also their own responses to the sick person. They face role changes as well as adjustments to progressing disability. These are demands in *addition* to the ordinary developmental tasks.

Understanding the Pressures of Change: Transitions are Never Easy

In illness, there is a fine line between independence and dependence. It is often healthy to become dependent because it permits others to do things to you and for you, that they would normally not have done. However in a marriage or a family, it is healthy to do as much as you can for yourself. MSer couples struggle to work out this contradiction while striving to keep their relationship intact.

To understand this problem in a new way, consider the life cycle in terms of transitions between stages, and interruptions to the steady growth of your relationship. How can you stop being an overbearing caretaker or a resentful, blaming patient? Seek to understand your problems, discuss options and strategies so that you can move beyond such a stagnated relationship.

Another benefit of the life cycle idea is that it widens your perspective. Instead of thinking only about the MS or the person with MS, you can include the whole family.

Table 12-1

THE STAGES OF THE FAMILY LIFE CYCLE

From: *The Family Life Cycle: A Framework for Family Therapy* by Elizabeth A. Carter and Monica McGoldrick. New York: Gardner Press (1980).

Family Life Cycle Stage	Emotional Process of Transition: Key Principles
1. Between families: The Unattached Young Adult	Accepting parent-offspring separation
2. The Joining of Families Through Marriage: The Newly Married Couple	Commitment to new system
3. The Family With Young Children	Accepting new members into the system
4. The Family With Adolescents	Increasing flexibility of family boundaries to include children's independence
5. Launching Children and Moving On	Accepting multitude of exits from and entries into family
6. The Family in Later Life	Accepting the shift of generational roles

Table 12-1. The family life cycle: One way to consider adaptations to multiple sclerosis in family systems. See text. Stages of family development and tasks for each stage are described.

The Family Life Cycle

Table 12-1 shows six stages in the life cycle of an ordinary family. The stages are listed in the first column, and attitude changes in the second. These are required if the family is to move on to the next stage.

Examine Table 12-1 and consider what additional tasks MS adds.

Stage 1: The Unattached Young Adult

If you are an unattached young adult and have MS, where do you *go*? The chart shows that the key emotional process is acceptance of separation between parent and young adult. Additional tasks of this time are the development of intimate relationships with others, finding a job, and development of different connections with the family. MS complicates these tasks. If you are sick, you can't be as independent as before. The previous pattern of protective parent—dependent child can again develop. This can prevent you from going out to work, making peer relationships and becoming a separate adult.

So what do you do? That depends on how disabled you are. The more control you have over your own care and daily tasks, the more independent you can feel. You may need to relearn job and relationship skills. In your new situation, you may want to discover how you can give to others. Much of the scrappiness of young disabled people is an expression of their effort to do just this. Families who take back a young disabled adult must also struggle with their own sadness about the MS.

Stages 2-3: Young Couples and Families With Young Children

Young couples make a commitment to their relationship and to their new family. When MS strikes, the tasks change. Perhaps the marital contract should be renegotiated. (Did I *really* mean for better or worse?) The couple needs to deal with grief and loss, and to understand MS as well as possible.

It is probably easier for couples who meet each other after MS is diagnosed. Then the contract between them is clear and open. There are, of course, the inevitable family struggles! Who does what? Who decides what? Who gives in? Which TV show do we watch? Answering these questions may form the basis for working out commitment. With MS in the picture, the balance can be more disrupted. The couple may fight over little things, when MS, grieving or resentment, are the real issues. We will discuss this more in a later section.

When children are born, there are new commitments: accepting the new baby, adjusting the marital system, taking on a parent role and realigning relationships with parents.

During this period, parents are frequently under stress. Young children drain both MSer and caretaker, and this can affect the marital balance. Exhaustion can cause sexual problems for both partners. The need for outside help may also lead to overinvolvment of the extended family. It is important for the couple to understand and discuss all these pressures. Children need a great deal of attention. So do the parents. Couples often ignore their own needs, and get caught in negative behavior patterns. They do too much, and then feel resentful toward the partner. In my work with such couples, I stress the importance of the couple relationship. I urge them to relearn how to care for each other, even while raising their children.

Stage 4: The Family with Adolescents
and
Stage 5: The Family Launching Children

As children get older, the chart shows that the family needs to become flexible first, to allow the children more independence, and second, to permit the adults to face their own mid-life issues. Increasing disability with MS may interfere with these needs. In MS families teens are expected to be more responsible. They may react by being totally irresponsible, by misbehaving, or by being too responsible. Peer group pressures may lead adolescents to deny the MS problems, to internalize their feelings, and to be depressed. Few adolescents are honest with their friends about MS. When the disease progresses, family depression may increase. As adolescent needs for possessions increase, financial pressures are more keenly felt.

It may not be as hard for MS families to launch their children, because as children leave, the burdens also decrease. The tasks connected with disability may make other illnesses, and even deaths less traumatic.

Stage 6: The Family in Later Life

The last period of the family occurs in later life. Old age increases physical burdens, but MSers are able to apply previous coping methods to aging and physical problems. This stage may thus be less of a transition for MS families.

RESOURCES: MATURITY, MEMORY, AND TIME

Because MSers are adults, they already possess strengths and abilities for dealing with MS. One person commented that he was grateful his MS brought him no pain. Another woman gained perspective from thinking that others were worse off than she. This point of view is the result of maturity. Normal growth allows a person to develop flexibility, to accept reality, and to compromise. Maturity enables one to learn new ways to solve problems, and to discover new pleasures.

Most MSers grew up as normal healthy people. Their memories can be an emotional resource to help them adjust to disability with a sense of integrity. One MSer developed a meditation exercise. Each morning, before she got out of bed, she imagined herself as a physically healthy person. Combined with relaxation, and possibly some spiritual meditation, such imaging can be learned and incorporated into the therapy for both MSer and care giver (2, 3, 14).

Memories provide stories to tell to children, about times when there was no MS. Such stories enrich a child's life and strengthen family ties.

Time is a third resource. Because MS takes time to develop, there is also time to adjust. There is time for family members to learn how weakness affects gait, time for families to learn to work together. Each episode teaches MSer and family a little more about what works and what does not. The ability to learn from each exacerbation can improve MS management.

RELIGIOUS FAITH AS A RESOURCE

Many MSers have written that their religious faith has been an important resource in dealing with MS. Religion offers help and guidance for resolving grief and lessening guilt.

Nancy Chaffee, an Episcopal Clergywoman who works with disabled people of all kinds, considers that suffering is part of our human condition. Suffering is real. It is the dark side of life. Rev. Chaffee emphasizes the need to acknowledge suffering and move beyond it, while still living with it. Society tends to deny suffering, while religion affirms it.

Rev. Chaffee, herself disabled, discovered that physical disability causes discomfort to other people. She learned that it was their problem, not hers. She learned slowly not to be ashamed of her disability, but to look beyond it to the gifts God had given her.

Grief and bitterness were strong in her own struggle with cerebral palsy. Grieving about disability needs to be done over and over again, she says. It is important to know that grief returns to people with chronic illness.

> "It is possible to find God in the midst of suffering," she said. "We tend to think God doesn't grieve with us. God grieves. We are not alone in suffering. We have permission to be angry at God for suffering. God can take it.
>
> "I contend that disability is a universal condition, rather than a particular condition. For centuries, the church focused on the sin, the sickness, or the shame of differentness. If we are to be a healing community, we must work toward healing, acceptance, and incorporating

diversity . . . . I am accepted and affirmed as a whole person, a person who is in the image of God. My limitations are accepted for what they are, more visible and slightly different from those of others (6)."

Other writers and MSers describe similar ideas, as they grapple with illness and disability. Frequently poetry, prayers, meditation provide a way to summon spiritual resources.

CHALLENGES OF MS

Maturity, memory, time, and religious faith are resources. MS also presents unique challenges. First, the diagnosis is not straightforward. That means that reality is not clearly defined. Fatigue, mild incoordination, and changes in emotional control are all physical manifestations of MS. They can be annoying, and may be misinterpreted by well meaning family members and MSers alike. Is it laziness or weakness? Is it pain or wimpiness? There is no easy answer. Acknowledge the ambiguity and complexity of MS symptoms, and expect that you will sometimes misinterpret them.

Unpredictability is another challenge. The uncertain course means that MSers and their families are never sure how long a remission or exacerbation will last. This can lead either to short-term planning only, or to no planning at all.

The move from fully functioning adult to patient, and from care giver to care receiver requires a major adjustment in a marriage or relationship. One study suggests that the hardest adjustments are those that remove us from work or family tasks: when a father cannot work or a mother care for the house and family (1).

Adjustments can be a challenge, or an insurmountable barrier. Children spoke graphically of the hopeless feeling they had when Dad quit his job, and of angry feelings when Mom wasn't there to go to school functions. Why could other fathers play with their children, certain that this could not happen to them?

For couples, the give and take becomes different with chronic illness. Frequently, a retreat toward isolation and withdrawal further complicates the change of roles. If a man with MS becomes depressed because he thinks he is unproductive, he may not realize that his spouse also needs emotional support. Couples who make the adjustment successfully confront these role changes openly.

It is vitally important during such role changes to acknowledge the grief and sadness of giving up an important role in life. Keep communication direct and open, and maintain the distinction between yourselves and your children. Expand your ability to tolerate your partner's foibles.

The sexual relationship presents a continuing challenge. As MS progresses, sensation and physical movement decrease. This is discussed in a later chapter. I introduce it here as a family challenge because sexual tensions, or sexual closeness and warmth between partners, can influence the emotional life of the whole family.

Depression in the MSer, discussed in Chapter 7, is also a common *family* reaction. In some families people take turns being depressed. In others, depression pervades the whole household. Most discussions with therapists or friends concentrate on MSers' responses to diagnosis and disability, but a more complete understanding of the process must include the family as well.

When you think about your family as a system you will realize that it is not only the MSer who reacts and adjusts, but everybody in the family. This may add to your perspective as you work out your own solutions within your MS family.

ATTITUDES OF OTHERS TOWARD MS: NOT YOUR PROBLEM

You and your MS family are not isolated. All the people you meet have to cope with the embodiment of MS. Studies show that physically healthy people have altered perceptions of disabled people. When interviewers were in wheelchairs, people were more positive and accommodating, and gave shorter interviews. They were less critical and confrontational than with interviewers who were not wheelchair-bound (10,11).

MSers tell stories of insensitive remarks, of being ignored, or of having someone be very friendly and then move quickly away. Just as you and your family need to adjust, so do others. Remember: Don't take responsibility for the discomfort of others. If you remind yourself that part of it is *their* problem, you may be able to go beyond the first reactions.

Self-Esteem and Disability: Also a Family Affair

Personal self-esteem, or the lack of it, affects our interaction with others and our attitudes toward life (4, 7, 15). Self-esteem begins early, with being held, cuddled and valued. MSers grow up as normal children, so most have received the nurturing that is basic to developing self-esteem. The experience of a normal childhood can be a rich resource for MSers who are parents, for it affirms their own children's worth. Whether or not you are disabled, you can still affirm your children in important ways. For example: "You have a right to be here. I recognize and respect your needs. You don't have to hurry." These are messages we give through touching, hugging, or with words. They are the messages we need to hear in infancy, and continue to throughout life. As children grow, they need affirmations for independence, for accomplishments, for thinking ability, for learning to do things, for growing up, and for growing away from us. In *Self-Esteem, A Family Affair*, Jean Isley Clark suggests that we give ourselves and others "strokes:" hugs, simple statements, looks of approval or other actions that increase self-esteem. In families the need for self-esteem and the need for food are of equal value. However, to affirm others, adults need to feel lovable and capable themselves. In their study, Matson and Brooks (13) found that MSers have a self concept similar to that of physically healthy people. They also observed that the longer a person has MS, the more his or her self concept improves.

Useful work is one important determinant of esteem among MSers. Important jobs include volunteering, church activities and family involvement. Counseling is helpful to many MSers when the self concept is assaulted by disability. Counseling is useful to spouses, children, and teens, when self-esteem is affected by the changes brought about by MS.

What can you do about self-esteem in your own family? Think carefully about the above affirmations. Try using them with those you love. Take care of your own self-esteem. Be aware that you cannot change fate, but you can change your attitude about fate. Each morning, try visualizing yourself as the person you're proud to be. Imagine how your partner and children look when they feel confident. Then try to keep that image with you as you interact with them. Self-esteem is indeed a family affair. Throughout our lives we can grow and improve our self image despite aging or disease.

REFERENCES:

1) Anthony, E. J.: Mutative Impact of Serious Illness in a Parent on Family Life. In: Anthony, E. J.; Koupernik, C.: *The Child in His Family*, Vol. 2. New York, Wiley and Sons, 1973.

2) Benson, H.: *The Relaxation Response*. New York, Avon Books, 1975.

3) Bloomfield, H.; Cain, M.; Jaffe, D.: *T. M.: Discovering Inner Energy and Overcoming Stress*. New York, Delacorte Press, 1975.

4) Briggs, D.: *Your Child's Self Esteem*. New York, Doubleday, 1975.

5) Carter, E. A.; Mc Goldrick, M., eds.: *The Family Life Cycle: A Framework for Family Therapy*. New York, Gardner, 1980.

6) Chaffee, N.: A Woman's Journey: Cerebral Palsy to Priesthood. *The Witness*. Vol. 68 No. 1, January, 1985.

7) Clark, J. I.: *Self Esteem: A Family Affair*. Minneapolis, Winston, 1978.

8) Erickson, E. H.: *Childhood and Society*. New York, Norton, 1963. Pages 247–274.

9) Glueckauf, R. L.; Quittner, A. L: Facing disability as a Young Adult: Psychological Issues and Approaches. In: Eisenberg, M. G.; Sutkin, L. C.; Jansen, M. A., eds.: *Chronic Illness, And Disability through the Life Span: Effects on Self and Family*. New York, Springer (Series on Rehabilitation, Vol. 4.) 1984. Chapter 8.

10) Kleck, R.: Physical Stigma and Nonverbal Cues Emitted in Face-to-Face Interaction. *Human Relations.* Vol. 21, No.1. Pages 19–28, 1968.

11) Kleck, R.; Ono, H.; Hastorf, A. H.: The Effects of Physical Deviance upon Face-to-Face Interaction. *Human Relations.* Vol. 19, No.4. Pages 425–436, 1966.

12) Levinson, D. J.: *Seasons of a Man's Life.* New York, Ballantine Books, 1979.

13) Matson, R.; Brooks, N.: Adjusting to Multiple Sclerosis, an Exploratory Study. in: *Social Science and Medicine.* Vol. 2. Pergamon Press, Ltd. 1977.

14) Mills, J.: *Coping with Stress: A Guide to Living.* New York, John Wiley & Sons, inc., 1982.

15) Satir, V.: *People Making.* Palo Alto, Science and Behavior Books, 1972.

16) Sheehy, G.: *Passages. Predictable Crises of Adult Life.* New York, Dutton, 1976.

Chapter 13
Marriage and MS
By Mitzi Wolf

How do you struggle? You hang on and let go. You love and joy in the thought that this is the best of all possible worlds....it hasn't been easy, but it's a fact that the finest steel is tempered in the hottest fire.

Verah Johnson
(Prologue)

We stay because of what we had before. People look at us with great romantic stares, but our relationship is like a yo-yo, up and down. When we talk about breaking up, we get scared of loneliness and isolation.

Marcia Fellows

There is such a meanness in our house now, such a lack of caring. We have no additional reserve of energy for each other. Our lives are taut with maintaining the balance to get through each day. There are no favors given. We thought ours was a pretty good marriage, but . . . when tested, when push came to shove, when better became worse, we really didn't fare so well at all. How disappointed we are in one another! (5)*

CHRONIC ILLNESS STRESSES MARRIAGE

MS itself does not make or break marriages, but chronic illness adds stress to marriage. The women above speak of the struggle of marriage in families with MS and other physical problems. Major role changes are required when one spouse becomes sick. Major adjustments occur in the marital balance during the course of MS. Both partners adjust to advancing disability. Power alignments change. Roles change. Sexual relationships change.

If one partner is sick and the other well, what difference does that make? Some couples find it makes very little difference. If the memory of "what we had before" is strong enough, couples continue their partnership in spite of physical disability. Some couples discover a strengthened relationship in disability. Most couples, however, do not find the role changes easy. We are more aware of our darker side when we confront illness. Anger and depression cannot be hidden away and forgotten. Each family deals with anger, depression and despair in unique ways.

> "I remember saying to Dick once that I was never cut out to be a nurse. This is not my calling!" His reply, "Well, I was never cut out to be a patient!" That shut me up. We have worked together at our unchosen vocations.
>
> Verah Johnson
> (Prologue)

---

* Note: References for this chapter may be found on page 245.

Flexibility and resilience are qualities that help relationships survive adversity. The most difficult role changes interfere with traditional roles: mother, wage earner, nurturer. These role changes affect everybody, and require several adjustment stages. First each person must experience the changed role. Then disarray and disorganization occur, as the change affects the life of the family. Then, there is a period of mourning, sadness and anger about this change. Last, the slow process of rebuilding the family around "unchosen vocations." Couples often have trouble as they work through role changes. The MSer is likely to be overwhelmed by grief and sadness. The caretaker spouse may not allow enough time to experience that sadness.

It becomes a major task to keep communication open during these transitions. Therapists help such a couple tell each other about their disappointment. In the opening quotation, Fern Kupfer wrote that they were disappointed in each other. Awareness does not eliminate the disappointment, but it is one step forward in abandoning despair. Once the couple have examined their disappointment and grief together, they can sometimes find a new starting point.

ADVANCING DISABILITY AND MARRIAGE

The same role changes and adjustments recur as disability advances. A father, who once cared for the children at home while his wife worked, developed increasing fatigue as the MS worsened. He slept while the children ran around the house and neighborhood. He and his wife struggled with their sadness about his illness, and with her resentment of the additional strains on her. She aired her resentment and shared her frustration directly with her partner. This lightened the burden for them both.

MS defines physical limits. The family encounters psychological and physical limits that are not as clear. Such limits are sometimes affected by the passage of time, by the acquisition of perspective, and by encouragement or discouragement from family members or other people.

There is a time to define your limits. If you need help with increasing disability, and your family is too stressed to help, you may benefit from outside help: concrete physical services or psychological support. You do not know in advance the extent of your physical and emotional reserves. It is important to know that there *are* limits. There are times we must say, "I can't."

FIGHTING FOR MARITAL SURVIVAL

Is it fair to fight with a spouse who is disabled? Successful couples fight and argue despite the illness. It clears the air if the issue is straightforward and if there is no feeling of guilt about being angry with someone in a wheelchair. During arguments, couples can work out compromises that help them deal with intimacy and distance. Fights get people moving. All of these are legitimate reasons. Here are some ideas about "fighting fairly" to help you evaluate your own style of fighting (1).

Anger is normal. But it is important to learn to express it in acceptable ways. We can all act a little nicer than we feel, but not much. Simple, non-blaming remarks like "I'm mad!" or "I'm in a bad mood today, so watch out!" give us and the other fellow a clear statement. When you are angry and can say it out loud, ask

240

yourself what the *real* issue is. For instance, it may *seem* that the children are excessively noisy today, when it's your spastic legs that are irksome. The children are handy scapegoats. If you discover the *real* issue, say it as clearly as you can.

The next step is very hard. *Listen* to what the other person says, then try to *repeat it back*. Filter it through your admittedly angry brain. "I hear you say I am feeling sorry for myself and taking it out on the kids." Or "I hear you say that I expect too much of you when you feel tired." Do not underestimate how hard it is to say such simple statements. It involves careful listening, and then judicious speaking when your anger wants release!

When you fight, concentrate on *one* point. Do not dredge up yesterday's issues, his or her mother's faults, insults. You can fight well if you follow these ground rules. *You* get to say your piece, then your partner. Both must listen. Once you have started this way, you can work toward compromise or stalemate, possibly toward an apology, or a change in behavior. Fights cause trouble when you do not know the *real* issue, or fail to limit yourself to one issue. Fights are destructive when you are deaf to the other person's complaint, or when you abandon the issue in order to hurt the other person, or attack the other person's personality.

One couple explored their pattern of fighting, and concluded that their arguments were useful for each to blow off steam. It also energized the MSer to do his morning exercises! He noted, "We do argue about the routine. I don't agree, but I usually end up doing what needs to be done." Their fight got the system moving.

Many of the nagging fights in MS families center around the frustrations of MS. If that is the issue, say it.

Be disappointed. Be sad for a while. However, some partners can't stand this. They are overwhelmed by the need to "get her out of her bad mood" or to "cheer him up." MSers can make a positive contribution to relationships if they help their partners learn the *real* issue, and relieve them of the job of cheerleader.

SEXUAL RELATIONSHIPS AND MS

Chapter 15, by Bernice Gottschalk and Mike Sarette, discusses sexual issues. Their discussion of their own experiences, of interviews with numerous MSers and their partners, and of the literature reflects the unique situation of couples and individuals who live with MS. Family issues further complicate sexual issues.

The adult resources of memory, imagination and fantasy can be useful to minimize the effects of MS on the sexual aspects of the relationship. Most MSers have a fund of memory of sexual experiences to draw upon in recreating their sexual relationships as the disease progresses. Sexual affirmation is important. Adults who have had relationships have had this affirmation. The arrival of children affirms our sexuality as well.

As MS progresses, couples will want to explore their new feelings and ideas about their sexual relationship. Experts can help.

Research suggests that sexual difficulty begins with the symptoms of MS itself. Fatigue, weakness, and sensory loss affect sexual desire. They appear just when both partners need every possible resource to nurture and comfort each other, and neither partner understands the trouble (2).

When the diagnosis of MS finally becomes certain, anger, frustration, denial, depression, and guilt affect both partners. None of these promotes a fulfilling sexual relationship. How can a couple readjust? Options for discussing sex are greater today. People are freer to express sexual preferences and behaviors. Increased knowledge and broader definitions of sexual expression give contemporary couples greater freedom in redefining their sexual relationships.

When should you seek professional help? An educational session with a sex therapist can provide some ideas to talk about. Indeed, it may be wise to consult a therapist *before* there is a crisis. Read the Chapter 15 to discover how other couples manage their relationships. Consider all issues: the role changes, communication, sexual relationships, and coping with progressing disability. They are the challenges. Talking about them won't eliminate them, but talking might provide options when things get difficult.

SEPARATION AND DIVORCE

Not all relationships succeed. What if you can't cope? A woman, whose husband was ill, paced up and down in my office, saying that she could put up with drinking and carousing, but not this! Eventually she left him. Terrible? I am sure she feels terrible. She just couldn't cope with illness. Her honesty may have been better for both her and her husband, than living together and hating each other. Separation in an MS family produces all the upsets of any separation, compounded by the guilt of leaving when things are bad. In such situations, find whatever support you can: individual counseling, religious help, MS groups, social support for all family members. If they can remain neutral, grandparents and other family members can often support children through marital breakups.

Like other kinds of grief, separation and divorce have their own stages. Kessler (4) lists seven stages, beginning with the first recognition of exaggerated marital discord. These stages are 1) disillusionment, 2) erosion, 3) detachment, 4) physical separation, 5) mourning, 6) second adolescence, and 7) hard work. If problems are aired and resolved at the stage of disillusionment, the second step, erosion of the relationship, may not occur. Following erosion, things appear normal but are not. Detachment is the period before physical separation. The tragedy of many marital breakups is that one partner is unaware, even when the partner is detaching. It is only at the time of actual physical separation, that many partners learn that the relationship is in trouble. After separation comes mourning, and then a second adolescence where new relationships are risked, often with underlying insecurity and lack of trust. Finally, there is the last stage, the hard work of being separated, divorced or reattached.

If you are separating or divorcing, look over this process, find out where you are and where your partner may be. If you are in the disillusionment stage, there is still time to talk, to seek help, to work at saving the relationship. It takes two people to make a marriage work. If one partner has become detached, it is difficult to reverse the process. Mourning is painful, and the feeling of being rejected by one's partner increases the grieving. In divorce, more than the relationship with the spouse is lost. Sometimes relationships with children, in-laws, and friends are sacrificed. For the abandoned partner, the grieving period can be prolonged. Kessler suggests that the last stage, hard work, makes it possible to come through the whole process and recover from the trauma of divorce.

HARD WORK

Relationships are never easy. Many people I see in my practice expect them to be simple. Some young couples move into partnerships expecting to receive, not to give. If you have been hurt, it may be difficult to give again in a new relationship and to learn to trust again. Framo (3) describes marriage as a "rhythmic epic, an insoluble power problem, and the one great human arena for growing and loving." All relationships are challenging. All need work, but usually, the work is worth the effort. MS adds just one more complication.

REFERENCES:

1) Bach, G. R.; Wyden, P.: *The Intimate Enemy*. New York, Avon Books, 1968.

2) Barrett, M.: *Sexuality and M.S.* Toronto, Multiple Sclerosis Society of Canada, 1977, page 1.

3) Framo, J.: *Object Relations View of Marriage and Marital Therapy*. Audio Tape Cassette Lecture, 1979.

4) Kessler, S.: *The American Way of Divorce: Prescription for Change*. Chicago, Nelson—Hall, 1975.

5) Kupfer, F.: *Before and After Zachariah*. New York, Delacorte, 1982, pp.101–102.

Chapter 14
Parents, Children and MS
By Mitzi Wolf

MS parents may become so involved in their own frustrations that the children feel isolated and confused. Each reacts differently to these feelings. One child may respond by being super-responsible, another by being the opposite. Some may want to run away. Most will worry about what their friends will say. When parents are upset, children may think that the parents are angry at *them*! They may even feel it is their fault that a parent is sick. Even though they are told otherwise, some children worry that they may catch MS, or that the MS parent may die soon.

One of a child's hardest jobs is to explain MS to friends. It is also hard to have to do extra chores, to stay home when friends go out, and watch non-disabled families play together. Children often feel upset when they see their MSer parent looking tired, sad or incapacitated. One young person spoke about losing hope when his father had to quit work. Until that point he had denied the reality of MS. Now he had to accept it.

In adapting to MS, everyone experiences loss of hope. Most finally accept reality, and begin again to hope. During this experience, children can be less isolated if their parents talk with them as they themselves learn to accept MS. By rejecting denial and accepting illness, MSers can be a model for their children.

CHILDREN COPE

Confronted with MS, children and teens tend to withdraw and deny. Parents can decrease their childrens' isolation by including them in the diagnostic process, by recognizing their withdrawal as normal and by utilizing peer groups. Teens and children of MS families can help *each other* to feel less isolated.

Parents should expect their children to cope in different ways. Children who have temper tantrums, sibling fights, and who stop talking and communicating with everyone cope negatively. They also tend to stay away from home, break rules, feel angry, and want to run away. Those who cope positively participate in school activities, sports, church and social activities. They turn to neighbors, deepen their friendships, and may seek counseling. Counseling sessions help children gain perspective on growing up in an MS family.

Adolescents are sensitive to the opinions of others. They yearn for acceptance by their peer group. Most teens find it difficult to discuss MS with their friends. They report two useful survival techniques, denial and leaving home. One boy told his friends that his dad had been in an auto accident!

PARENTING AND MS

"Children need encouragement, as a plant needs water, and parents need the courage to be imperfect."
Rudolph Dreikurs
Child development has its own cycle, and its own

issues and stresses. The more parents know about MS, the more objective they can be. They can use their knowledge to help their children and themselves. How? By reducing their feeling of guilt about having a home with a disabled family member.

Parents can work at being responsible for their own attitudes. When parents become aware of what children are feeling, they can help them talk about those feelings. I have already suggested that MSers may help children in the initial stages, by expressing their own awareness of denial, anger and frustration. Children are reassured when an MSer parent admits to anger about the MS. It helps to say that the anger has nothing to do with the child. The MSer parent can be clear about these feelings. Children do not need to be shielded from the sadness and frustration of illness. In manageable doses, real feelings and real experiences prepare children for life.

PARENTING AS A SKILL

Dreikurs's ideas might form the basis for parent study groups, or MS support groups to help MSers and spouses learn to understand their children's behavior. Members of the group can support and encourage one another in the complicated job of being a parent.

We all need to belong. Children's behavior can be understood as a way to belong, as a search for attention, approval, and affection. If children feel they belong, their behavior is more likely to be cooperative and positive. If they feel excluded, they often become discouraged and misbehave. The child's place in the family constellation is a powerful determinant of personality development. The oldest is usually domineering, but the most responsible. The middle child is often more likable and less reliable. The youngest is babied, and frequently is very different from the rest (3,4);*. Children in the same family do not have the same experiences, no matter how strongly parents insist they treat them similarly.

Therefore, children from one family will react differently to illness, to growing up, as well as to other challenges. This continues to surprise parents. However, if a family is prepared for these differences, each child has more freedom to find his own best way.

DEALING WITH MISBEHAVIOR

Dealing with children's behavior and misbehavior is never simple. MS makes it even more complex. Here are some guidelines. If they interest you, read Dreikurs' books, listed at the end of this chapter (1, 2, 3,).

Your *first* reaction to a child's misbehavior may not be your best reaction. There are reasons why children do things. Sometimes they are wrong. Often they misunderstand how to get what they want. If your child misbehaves, step back. Try to understand why he is misbehaving. Then plan a reaction that will teach him something useful.

Dreikurs suggests that parents need to be uninvolved emotionally to discipline effectively. Discipline can become a logical outcome of specific misbehavior. By not protecting a child from the natural consequences of the act, a parent hopes to teach a child two things: not to misbehave, and to take responsibility for his own ac-

---

* Note: References for this chapter may be found on page 252 and 253.

tions. Dreikurs suggests giving children constant encouragement to behave positively. By offering acceptance and affirmation, parents foster self-esteem. Consider the ideas about affirmation in Chapter 12, on family relationships (1).

The physically healthy parent in the MS family may be responsible for the physical care and discipline of the children. However, it is wise for both parents to share their parenting, even when one is physically disabled. Family meetings and discussions can incorporate their ideas about parenting. Including the MSer parent in discussions with the child assures him that decisions are made by *both* parents. In this way, the idea of parents as a team can be sustained, and can benefit parents *and* children.

ADOLESCENCE

Adolescence is a time when *all* parent-teen relationships are strained. Adolescents must grow up and discover who they are. They must become independent and develop a sexual identity. Few of us do this gracefully. MS makes this transition even more difficult for teenagers and their parents. Some teens stay away from home. Some get absorbed in school or peer activities. Some deny the family situation to friends. Some misbehave, while others become overresponsible. Teenage anxiety is compounded by family concerns. This state of mind leads teenagers to bounce higher and fall lower as they grow.

Parents who survive their adolescents do so by taking care of themselves and supporting each other emotionally. They approve little, tolerate much, and rely on a good sense of humor! Whenever possible, parents give the teenager the clear message that they are in charge. When rebellion occurs, natural consequences can help teenagers learn their limits and parents define the boundaries of their parenting job.

Some teenagers curse the family and blow off steam at home. The same young person may conform in other relationships. Logical consequences, discussed as a method of dealing with misbehavior in younger children, are also applicable to teens. When teens fail to perform family tasks, parents can respond by being unavailable for rides or favors.

In the family we can be both our best and our worst. The need to express fury can be acknowledged and perhaps even encouraged. MSers need to explode and so do their spouses and children. The trick is to know how much to explode, how to do it without blaming, and how to end the explosion. Perhaps a smile, a gesture, a kiss, or just a look can help the rest of the family move on. In the safety of the family we can start over again, and again, and again.

TROUBLES IN THE FAMILY

Some families, with or without MS, can discuss problems together and work things out. Others cannot. These three chapters on family and parent relationships highlight the strengths and the potential weaknesses in MS families. When difficulties develop in family life, the first resource is the family itself. When that is not enough, you may wish to pursue professional counseling. If you do need help, go early. Do not wait until someone threatens to leave, or an insurmountable crisis occurs. Deep wounds heal slowly.

Most MSers who need treatment, need treatment as

families, not individually. Family therapists come from many disciplines: psychiatry, social work, psychology, marriage and family counseling and pastoral counseling. Just as you search for quality in a physician, search for quality in a family counselor. Friends, the local MS Chapter, your physician, minister or community resource agency may be able to recommend individuals or agencies that can best address your needs.

AFTERTHOUGHT

There are many ways to raise children, as a trip to your nearest bookstore will show. In this chapter, I have presented a democratic approach—to a point. I always recommend that parents remain in charge.

One of our editors, a mother of three, questioned the practical application of this theory. She runs her family as a "loving dictatorship" and feels that works for her. I agree that parents should be the ultimate rule makers and enforcers, even in the Dreikurs approach. Leadership rests with the parents. Children need adults who care enough to make rules that organize their world, and who define limits that foster security.

Parenting is a delicate balance of giving and withholding, of holding close and letting go. The unique personality of each family member requires the family unit to be adaptable. Perhaps you can fit ideas from this chapter into your own family. But like our editor above, if your approach works, don't change it unless you are sure you understand what you are doing.

REFERENCES:

1) Clark, J. I.: *Self-Esteem: A Family Affair.* Minneapolis: Winston Press, 1978, page 263.

2) Dreikurs, R.; Cassel, P.: *Discipline Without Tears.* New York: Hawthorn Books, 1972.

3) Dreikurs, R.: Grey, L.: *A Parent's Guide to Child Discipline.* New York: Hawthorn Books, 1970.

4) Dreikurs, R.; Stoltz, V.: *Children: The Challenge.* New York: Hawthorn Books, 1964.

Chapter 15

Sexual Enhancement for MSers and Partners

By Bernice Gottschalk and Mike Sarette

For Mark

How can you love me?
Ugly,
That's what I see in me.
But you do!

Insanity!
I need you. I need your hugs, your love,
Your laughter.
You enrich my life!

Are you right, and I wrong?
Am I worth loving despite MS?
From heaven and earth I am bombarded with
Yes!

Transformation! I learn again
To love myself.

Bonnie Johannes
May, 1984

SEXUALITY IS MORE THAN SEX

All of us are sexual, whether or not we express our sexuality in the ways commonly thought of as "sex." MS changes the way we experience our bodies and challenges previous definitions of ourselves. Small wonder that it can have a profound effect on our sexuality. In addition, MS can interfere with sensation, movement, erection, lubrication or orgasm.

Sex is one way we express love and caring for another person, and one way we care for ourselves. Sex is fun. Sex is soft touches, hugs and feeling warmly close to your partner. Sometimes sex includes intercourse. Sometimes it leads to orgasm. Sometimes, even to babies. But none of these is *essential* to the enjoyment of sexual experiences.

Our society views sex as a dessert, not an integral part of the meal of life. Because of this, you may tolerate sexual dysfunction while you fight hard against other kinds of disability. We think a good sex life *is* worth fighting for. We have gathered ideas to help you and your partner toward a loving and fulfilling sexual life— despite MS.

Some MSers find that sex helps them continue to feel good about their bodies. You may be able to give pleasure by holding and hugging and touching. Sometimes love means bringing your partner to orgasm, even though you cannot give in other physical ways. Enjoy your body! Focus on the good feelings you experience, not on your losses.

YOU HAVE CHOICES

We hope you will find this chapter useful for the enjoyment of your body and your intimate relationships, even if you sometimes respond: "that's not for me!" Some people choose to avoid sex altogether. Some MSers feel it's easier to live without sex than to spend time and energy thinking about and working at sexual activities that are only marginally enjoyable. There is no rule that says you *must* have sex to live a happy life.

Some readers may feel that discussion of sexual activities is distasteful or wrong because of religious or moral beliefs. If you are interested in new ideas for retaining sexual enjoyment, but are uncertain about the views of your faith, consult a sympathetic member of the clergy.

COMMUNICATION IS VITAL, SO SPEAK YOUR FEELINGS

Keep talking with your partner! It is one of the most important things you both can do to prevent sexual crippling. Most of us do not discuss sex. We whisper. We giggle. Sometimes we brag. In our culture, men learn that good lovers automatically know how to please their partners. Women learn that men are frail creatures whose egos shrivel at any hint for improvement. Instead of talking, many couples turn to mind reading, and that usually doesn't work.

If you want your partner to know what you feel, *say it*. It's not always easy. No one wants to hurt a partner's feelings. But you will not necessarily hurt someone when you say you are frustrated or uncomfortable. For example, partners of men with erectile problems often fear they are at fault. It is *reassuring* to tell her that you still love her and are still turned on by her, but the signals aren't getting through to your penis. It may be equally reassuring for you to know that she's frustrated too, but she still thinks you're wonderful. You then have a problem to work on together, not a continuing source of blame and embarrassment between you.

If you have sensory loss, you both need to know it so you can discover what feels good now. Maybe it's scary to be touched where it's numb. Perhaps you shy away because similar touches have been unpredictably painful. Maybe your bladder has been acting up, and you are afraid of what might happen if you get carried away. It's better for your partner to know these things, than to wonder if you are disinterested.

If you are too tired for sex, but you would still like to be held until you fall asleep, say so. When you say "No," say whether you mean "See you next week," or "Wake me in an hour and we'll see!" It's possible to begin talking about sex now, even if you never did before. You may find that improved sexual intimacy helps your relationship in other areas too. Set aside a special quiet time for conversation. Hold each other if you like, but agree that this time the focus will be verbal, not physical. Talking *about* sex *during* sex detracts from both the talking and the sex.

Accentuate the Positive

It is easy to respond to: "I like it when you stroke my thighs gently," or "It really turns me on when you make the first move. "It's not so nice to hear: "Stop pinching me!" or "I'm sick of always having to be the one to start things." Tell your partner how you feel, but don't assign blame. "It hurts when you bite my nipples" is generally more effective than "You callous brute!"

Practice talking about your feelings and experiences. Take turns talking while the other listens. As you listen, you may discover that your assumptions about your partner's thoughts and feelings were completely wrong!

Perhaps there were times when you both wanted to stop and go to sleep, but you pressed on with increasing frustration because each was afraid of letting the other down. Maybe your partner thinks you don't like to kiss, when it's just that you need to come up for air. You might even discover that you'd both like to make love under the lilacs, but were afraid to be the first to mention it.

Learning new skills takes time, especially the skill of talking about this private part of life. At first you will both be uncomfortable. Use your shared discomfort to bring you together.

YOUR MIND IS THE SEXIEST PART OF YOU

What you do with your body is only part of sex. Your arousal, your enjoyment, and the depth of sharing with your partner depend in large part on what's going on in your head. Many people enjoy reading romantic or erotic books, looking at sexy pictures, or delighting in their own fantasies. These activities can be enjoyed alone or with a partner. They can be highly pleasurable *whether or not* they result in physical arousal. People sometimes fantasize about situations and sexual acts that would turn them off in real life. If your fantasies shock you, do not be alarmed. Fantasies are not reality!

Some couples who no longer participate in vigorous sex enjoy remembering "times when" together. These memories contribute to closeness and add a spark to everyday life. Through memories love remains, even though it is expressed in different ways.

ORGASM IS NOT THE ONLY PURPOSE OF SEX

If the only aim is orgasm, and orgasm won't come, sex can be more of a trial than a joy. But orgasm need not be your aim. The warm closeness of your partner's body and your shared pleasure in fulfillment can be enough. Most people like to be touched and fondled. Most can enjoy intercourse without having an orgasm.

Orgasm occurs in the mind. Sometimes the body participates too, as when a man ejaculates or a woman's vagina contracts rhythmically. But it is not necessary to be able to feel your genitals and it is unnecessary to ejaculate in order to experience an orgasm. Some men and women with complete loss of sensation below the nipples perceive and enjoy a sexual climax. They say it is different from previous experiences, but no less satisfying.

The Joy of Cuddling

Lie quietly. Hold each other's naked bodies. Appreciate each other and the flow of energy between you. It is one of the most intensely joyous, mutually affirming things you can do. If you read Ann Landers regularly, you know how many people cry out for this kind of love. They have not yet learned to cuddle. Sadly, many MSers stop cuddling when they find that sex doesn't work as it used to. They are afraid to start something they can't finish.

Cuddling can be serious or frivolous. You can comfort your partner when she's sad or giggle with him when things are funny. You can huddle together, waiting for the alarm to ring, or fall asleep like nestled spoons. Cuddling *can* lead to other things, but it doesn't have to.

EXPLORATION AND RELEARNING

Each time the MS changes, MSers need to rediscover their own bodies. You may find new means to satisfaction that can replace much of what you've lost. Some people with numbness below a certain point (called a sensory level, see page 308) find that their skin is particularly sensitive just above the numb area. This becomes a new erogenous zone.

Masturbation

If you want sex when your partner is too tired, if you need to learn what feels good, if you'd rather give pleasure to yourself than go to bed with someone you don't know well, then masturbate. One woman even reported that masturbation helps relieve her abdominal spasms.

There are many ways to masturbate. If sensory loss or incoordination interfere with a previous method, experiment. Take time to re-explore your whole body, not just your genitals. Try different strokes and different rhythms. Create a sensuous environment with music, lights, and textures. Look at romantic or explicit books and pictures. You may be pleasantly surprised at how much you still enjoy! A water soluble lubricant (such as K-Y® jelly, available at any pharmacy) can enhance pleasure and ease movement. Men may prefer baby oil, which does not evaporate. Women should avoid oily lubricants, which can promote vaginal or bladder infection. A vibrator can help if your hands get too tired or you need to intensify sensation.

Although masturbation is often pleasant without orgasm, some people find that masturbation is the surest route to orgasm. Many women have never masturbated.

If you'd like to try, but are unsure how to begin, Barbach's book, *For Yourself,* (3)* has many helpful suggestions.

Sensate Focus, A Way to Explore Each Other

Masters and Johnson (6) devised a technique often used in sex therapy, called "sensate focus." They found that if there is no pressure to perform, people can more easily concentrate on getting and giving pleasure. First, explore your own body. Then set aside time to explore each other's bodies. Decide *beforehand* not to let your exploration lead to intercourse or orgasm. Take turns touching each other. Vary where you touch and how you touch. Touch softly, then firmly, using your hands and other parts of you. Try short flicks and long continuous caresses. Use your imagination!

During sensate focus exercises, the person being pleasured concentrates completely on the touches and the feelings they arouse. Report to your partner what feels especially good and what does not. Take time to explore each other thoroughly. Remember that your genitals are only one part of you. Pay the most attention to the rest of your body. Discover how much pleasure you can experience! Plan to repeat this exercise in the future. Different touches may feel better next time. Additional exercises for sensory awareness are discussed in the books by Barbach (2, 3) and Zilbergeld (12).

Timing

Among able-bodied people, women are usually slower than men to become aroused. MSers often need

---

* Note: References for this chapter may be found on page 278.

more stimulation than their partners. Partners sometimes ignore their own natural pace in order to concentrate on what works for the MSer. For example, the partner of a man with erectile problems may feel she must rush into intercourse if he is ready, even though she is not. One woman told us she deals with this by using a lubricant for intercourse and masturbating in her husband's arms afterwards. That way she doesn't feel hurried, and can enjoy both the intercourse and her own orgasm.

Explore together to find the best timing for each of you. Approach the problem in the spirit of adventure. Sometimes things won't work out quite as planned. Have fun anyway, and learn more next time.

Sexual Aids

Vibrators are useful sexual aids for many people. They help weak or uncoordinated hands to masturbate successfully and to give pleasure to a partner. Vibrators can help those with numbness find greater satisfaction, but they are not for everyone. One MSer told us he doesn't like vibrators even though they enhance his erection. When he uses one, he ejaculates so rapidly that neither he nor his partner have enough time for enjoyment.

Catalogues of vibrators and other sexual aids are available (4, 9). You can also buy some types of vibrators, sold for "muscle relaxation," at discount stores and drugstores.

Other traditional erotic props can help MSers too. Mirrors (not *necessarily* on the ceiling) let you see what your partner is doing even if you can't feel. Waterbeds provide maximum motion with minimal effort and can make some otherwise uncomfortable positions pleasant.

Waterbed temperature can be controlled for comfortable cuddling in all seasons. Some people find waterbeds hard to get into and out of, but the soft sided ones pose less of a problem.

SEXUAL PROBLEMS OF MSers

In a recent study of people with MS, Valleroy and Kraft (8) found that three-quarters of the men and over half the women admitted to sexual difficulties. Among men, the most common complaint was getting or maintaining an erection. Women complained most frequently of fatigue. Other problems reported by men and women alike included altered or diminished sensation, difficulty achieving orgasm and decreased interest in sex. Ten percent indicated their partner as the major sexual problem. MSers with all degrees of disability reported sexual difficulties. Spasticity, weakness and bladder dysfunction interfere with sexual expression. Some MSers report no sexual problems even though they have these and many other MS symptoms.

Most MSers experience days of improved strength, better bladder control or lessened fatigue. There are also days when *everything* goes wrong. Good days and bad days occur in the sexual area too. On a bad day a man may not trust his erection. MSers of either sex may be unable to respond. Fatigue may interfere. Sex may be more irritating than enjoyable.

Sexual problems are common in the general population, too. Look in any bookstore. See how many of the volumes propose to improve the reader's sex life. If everyone had great sex, would there be so many books?

Do you think that "real sex" consists only of intercourse in the missionary position? Many people whose disability prevents them from having "standard" intercourse, nevertheless enjoy a degree of warmth, closeness, and even orgasmic satisfaction that would be the envy of many able-bodied people if only they knew!

Fatigue

Able-bodied people may also feel too tired for sex. But for MSers, exhaustion is a *major* source of frustration. It helps to plan sex (Make a date!) for a time or a day when you are usually more energetic. Sometimes it's fun to lie back, relax, and let your partner take over. Some other time, when you're more rested, you can return the favor. If you are tired, but you want to have intercourse, try a side by side position (either facing each other, or with the man behind the woman). These positions may prove less strenuous.

One woman told us she has great difficulty walking for at least an hour after intercourse. Because she now expects it, she is no longer alarmed. The enjoyment she gets from sex is worth the trouble.

If you are exhausted, even passive fondling may be too much. There's nothing wrong with saying no. "No" doesn't have to mean "never." Your partner can masturbate, or decide that the wait will make things better next time.

Lubrication

Some women MSers do not lubricate as readily or as fully as they once did, even though they feel ready for intercourse. Fortunately, it's easier to make up for this than for lack of an erection. Water soluble lubricating jelly (such as KY® Jelly) or contraceptive foam or jelly works well. Some people solve the problem with the premoistening that oral stimulation provides. Do *not* use water repellent vaseline, which might promote infection.

Erectile Problems

When erectile problems occur early, especially before diagnosis, people often look for psychological causes. Even after diagnosis, many MSers don't realize that *they are not to blame* for a reluctant penis.

Erectile difficulties are common among MSers. Some men never get an erection. More frequently, erections are fleeting or only semi-hard. Some men require a great deal of manual or oral stimulation to become erect. Formerly lovemaking may have involved more attention to a *partner's* arousal. Now they must focus longer and more intensely on themselves. Sometimes a vibrator helps men, just as it does women. Erectile dysfunction can come and go, like any other MS symptom.

Fantasy May Work Better than Direct Stimulation

Erection is controlled by several different pathways in the brain and spinal cord. (See pages 322–324.) Even if you don't respond well to direct stimulation you may become aroused through fantasy. Look at sexy pictures. Read racy novels. Remember sexy events. Experiment to see what works for you!

"Stuffing:" A Technique to Aid Intercourse

It *is* possible to have intercourse with a partial erection. It usually works best with the woman on top. She can use her hands to put her partner's penis inside her and can control her movements so it stays there. This can be pleasant whether or not it leads to orgasm. There is even a technical term used by sex therapists for this maneuver: "stuffing!" Some couples find they need extra lubrication in order for the man with a softer erection to enter. Saliva, K-Y® Jelly, and contraceptive foam or jelly all work well.

Don't Despair

Some men feel worthless if they can't have an erection. You may not understand why your partner still loves and wants you. You may not believe her when she says she does!

We talked to several couples who had struggled with this problem. Some husbands told their wives to have an affair or get a divorce. Others became jealous of their wives' male friends and acquaintances, suspecting affairs where none existed. Wives who were genuinely satisfied and in love with their husbands felt bitter and puzzled about this sudden lack of trust. Both members of the couple hurt badly. But reassurance sometimes made things worse.

If this describes your situation, you are not alone. You are probably reacting to this disease and its impotence, not to defects in each other's character. Rethink your ideas about the nature of manhood. Remember that men can fall to the depths of despair at impotence, and help each other with these feelings.

Intercourse is not the only means to sexual pleasure! You can be a warm, masculine, satisfying lover without an erect penis. Your partner wants *you*, not just old-fashioned sex. Read Zilbergeld's (10) book on male sexuality. Contact a therapist who specializes in family and marital counseling if you have trouble working this through by yourselves.

SEXUAL IMPLICATIONS OF OTHER MS SYMPTOMS

Bladder and Bowel Problems

Bladder and bowel problems interfere with sexual relationships. Many people become so concerned about a possible accident that they can't relax enough to enjoy. Learn everything you can about bowel and bladder management. (See Chapters 5 and 6.) Empty your bladder as completely as possible before sex. Talk with your partner about the possibility of an accident, to make its actual occurrence less traumatic. Some people feel more comfortable lying on a towel, or using a rubber sheet. Then if things go awry, there is less hassle to a bedding change. Side by side positions or positions with the MSer on top are safer because they place less pressure on the bladder.

For one woman we interviewed, rushing to the bathroom in the middle of sexual activity is a major annoyance. She and her partner find it best not to try to pick up where they were interrupted. They go back a few steps to rekindle passion.

If your partner usually helps with toileting or bladder and bowel care, you may find it hard to think of each other as sexual people. Need for these activities just before sex adds to the problem. Some people are quite comfortable switching from one role to the other, and make the physical closeness of care activities part of the loving attention of their sexuality. Others have more difficulty feeling sexy in those circumstances. Sometimes it helps to change the mood. Put on a negligee or sexy pajamas. Turn on the red light. Play romantic music. Then you can feel like a lover, not a patient or a nurse.

Indwelling Catheters

Indwelling catheters pose an interesting logistical challenge. Women can tape the catheter to the abdomen and proceed as usual. Some men fold the catheter back over the penis and put on a condom. This might hurt if you have feeling in your penis. It might prove inadequate if you need intense stimulation to maintain your erection. Some people simply remove the catheter, and then reinsert it after sex.

Spasticity

Severe spasticity makes it hard to separate the thighs. This makes intercourse difficult or impossible. Adjust the timing of your antispastic medication (See Chapter 4.) so you can have floppy legs when you have sex. It may help to have your partner gently exercise your legs. This exercise could even become part of foreplay. If despite everything you remain spastic, choose a position that requires minimal leg separation. A side-to-side position, with the man behind the woman, is often the easiest.

One man said that the approach of orgasm brings on painful leg spasms. He finds it helpful to push against the footboard (or headboard) of the bed with his toes, in order to release the spasms while continuing intercourse.

Depression

Depression quenches passion and destroys performance. Because depression takes the joy and spirit out of life, partners of depressed people may find them less attractive. Get the depression treated. (See Chapter 7.)

Your sexual function may improve considerably, and you will be better able to handle those problems that remain.

YOUR SEXUAL PROBLEMS MAY NOT ALL BE CAUSED BY MS

Other Illnesses and Medications Can Affect Your Sex Life

Other diseases, most commonly diabetes, can lead to erectile dysfunction. Some blood pressure medications are notorious for this side effect. Alcohol impairs sexual performance. Antidepressants sometimes interfere with sexual function. Many other drugs have been reported to affect desire, arousal, or satisfaction for some people. If you suspect that your medication has affected your sexual function, tell your doctor. There may be alternative treatments.

Anxiety Interferes

Anxiety interferes with anyone's sex life. Failed erection or loss of enjoyment worsen anxiety. This often leads to an expectation of failure. You may have regained lost sexual function after treatment of depression or recovery from an MS attack, but not even know it because of a self-fullfilling prophesy of failure! See the section on "sensate focus." (page 261) Read the books by Barbach (2, 3) and Zilbergeld, (11) for ideas that may enhance sexual responsiveness, and minimize anxiety.

Look at Your Relationship

Many times MS is only *part* of the problem. Sometimes sexual dysfunction is secondary to other problems between partners, or to other problems in life.

If you need help sorting these things out, consult a family and marital counselor, professional sex therapist or a urologist who specializes in sexual dysfunction. Ask your doctor for a referral. Write to the American Association of Sex Educators, Counselors and Therapists for a list of certified sex therapists in your state (1).

People are often embarrassed about seeking outside help for personal problems. Partners may feel disloyal when they reveal sexual problems to an outsider. A good counselor can help you through your discomfort as you explore your concerns together.

SPECIAL CONCERNS OF SINGLE MSers

Many singles have trouble finding partners. If you can't get out of the house, if the local mixing spots are all up three flights of stairs, if you met your last two girl friends hang gliding and you can't hang glide anymore —the problem is worse. It takes energy to develop new interests. It requires planning and persistence to participate. Sometimes it seems like too much trouble to work so hard just to meet people or even to find something that's fun to do. You are the only one who can decide if it's worth it to you.

Some MSers decide not to seek a sexual partner. They choose abstinence or masturbation. They develop rewarding nonsexual friendships.

If MS contributed to the break-up of a relationship, MSers wonder how they can trust the next person not to leave, too. Even if you have not been abandoned, you might hesitate to commit yourself to a willing partner because you fear eventual disappointment. You may need to take more time now, to test out the relationship and feel secure, than you would have before you got MS.

What to Tell a Partner

MSers sometimes worry about what to tell potential partners. Nobody wants to shout from the housetops: "I have MS!" but sometimes it is deceitful to be silent. Some partners *will* leave when you tell them. Such people probably could not have stood the pressure of MS anyway, and it is best for both of you to discover it early. Others will pay less attention to your disease than to all your other attributes.

There are no easy answers. But most people can learn to talk about MS honestly and with self-acceptance. A new partner needs information, just as you did when you were first told you had MS. Give your friend this book. Talk about MS, and how it has affected your life. If you have exacerbations and remissions, mention them. Discuss the variations of day-to-day energy levels that are *not* exacerbations. Otherwise your friend may panic when you are weaker than usual. If you have already discussed bladder problems, your friend won't wonder why you keep leaving the room. As your relationship develops, your friend can accompany you on a visit to the doctor, and meet other MSer couples with you.

One MSer stressed the importance of talking about potential sexual problems with a new partner beforehand, rather than just hoping for the best. That way it's less likely there will be unpleasant surprises.

Some Thoughts for Prospective Partners

If you are the potential partner of an MSer, you have undoubtedly heard some very scary things. They're scary to MSers too. You may wonder whether you can manage long term involvement with a disabled person, or whether you can stand to watch worsening disability.

You probably wonder if you have the strength and determination to carry through.

But have you worried whether you have enough laziness and selfishness to do a really *good* job? These qualities are also important for a successful relationship. You will need most of your laziness and much of your selfishness just to keep from doing things for your partner that he or she can do alone. Sometimes you will need them to let your partner take care of *you*.

Friends and relatives may tell you you're crazy to get involved with an MSer. (*Some* would say it if you planned to marry a healthy, handsome, considerate millionaire!) Others are genuinely concerned for your future happiness. Tell them the wonderful things about your relationship. It may help.

When you choose to love someone with MS, you accept more uncertainty in your life. You may try to prepare for the future from the beginning. You do face one hazard as a result. If your partner becomes severely disabled, you will feel bad, but you may tell yourself you have no *right* to feel that way, because you knew all along what you were in for. Nonsense! Of course you have a right to feel sad, angry and scared, just as your partner does. If you acknowledge that right you will be better able to help each other. Read Verah Johnson's Prologue to this book!

SPECIAL CONCERNS OF GAY AND LESBIAN MSers

In this society both disabled *and* gay people experience prejudice, so gay and lesbian MSers face a double stigma. Lesbian and gay MSers may feel they don't fit in with predominantly heterosexual groups of disabled people or with gay groups that are predominantly able-bodied. A lesbian or a gay man in an MS support group may hesitate to come out. Gay and lesbian organizations may meet in inaccessible places. Some gay and lesbian groups emphasize physical fitness and active participation in sports. Disability can prevent you from meeting friends and potential partners who share your sexual preferences.

On the other hand, lesbians and gays who have come to grips with their sexual orientation often have a healthier attitude toward sex than people who have never been forced to confront their sexuality. A gay psychologist friend contributed the following thoughts: "Gays may be more willing to talk about sex and to try alternative sexual techniques. Many gays have learned that self-esteem and personal fulfillment do not depend on living up to society's expectations. Although some gay men and lesbians prefer a variety of sexual partners, others prefer a long term relationship. It is important to recognize that these can endure despite illness and disability. The bond between lovers can be strengthened by the shared experience of extended illness." In some cities, disabled gay men and lesbians have formed groups for mutual support. If there is no such group in your community, start one with friends and invite others to join. Announce your meetings in the local MS newsletter as well as in lesbian/gay newspapers. The National Gay Task Force crisis line, (4) can inform you of existing groups in your state. Members of the Minneapolis Support Group for Lesbians and Gays with Disability (7) are willing to correspond with readers who want information and support.

EXPLOITATION

MSers are sometimes exploited in sexual relationships. Exploitation takes many forms—being forced into a relationship from fear of abandonment, being forced to do things that feel wrong, being treated badly by a partner who knows you cannot fight back, being paid money for sex by a partner as a token of disdain.

Sometimes able-bodied partners are exploited. They allow feelings of guilt about leaving a disabled partner, or economic dependence, to keep them in a destructive relationship.

In a relationship of equals, both partners defer to the other's wishes. Some sexual activities may be especially pleasurable to one, but not to the other. They share each other's pleasure, knowing that at other times things will go the other way. Neither partner feels coerced, and both have a right to individual preferences. When you are exploited, there is no such mutuality. The message is that the exploiter is free to leave at any time, and must be appeased at any cost. The message is also that no one else would be interested in you, or would be willing to put up with your MS.

Exploitation is possible only if you believe these messages. If *you* don't think you're worth much, someone else can take advantage of you. MS does not diminish your value as a person! No one has a right to humiliate you, nor to physically abuse you.

If you are being abused or exploited, and don't know how to escape, call a local family service agency, mental health clinic, health department, or social service department. Someone can arrange to see you, even if transportation is difficult. If the situation becomes dangerous rather than merely uncomfortable, call the abused person's hot line, if there is one in your state, or call the police.

KEEP US INFORMED!

Thanks to everyone who responded to our letters and answered our questions. We are especially grateful to the MS group in Nashville, Tennessee, who recorded their discussions and allowed us to use their tapes.

We need to learn more for future editions of this book. Write to us if you have learned techniques that help to overcome sexual problems, or if you have other information we should use.

FURTHER RESOURCES AND BOOKS TO READ

Sexual Attitude Reassessment Seminars (SARS)

These workshops are useful for some people. Seminars are usually scheduled for several days or a weekend. Films are shown and discussion groups formed to help people explore new sexual options in a nonthreatening environment. Many SARS are specifically designed for disabled people, their partners, and professionals.

To learn about SARS in your area, contact your hospital social work department, independent living center, or MS chapter.

Books on Sexuality

The books listed below contain information about sex, sexuality, and ways to improve sexual function despite disability. Some are written primarily for the general public, some for disabled people. Read and discuss them with your partner. They can help with communication, and might even turn you on. Enjoy!

Barbach, L.: *For Yourself: the Fulfillment of Female Sexuality.* New York, Signet, 1975.($2.95)
Helps women learn about their sexual functioning, to achieve orgasm. Includes exercises for self awareness and masturbation.

Barrett, M.: *Sexuality and Multiple Sclerosis.* Revised 1982. Available free from: National Multiple Sclerosis Society, 205 E. 42nd St., New York, NY 10017, or your local MS chapter. A review of MS-related sexual problems and options.

Becker, E.: *Female Sexuality Following Spinal Cord Injury.* Bloomington, Cheever Publishing (Accent Press), 1978. ($10.95)
This book is about women who are paralyzed after injuries. It consists of a series of interviews in which women talk about their feelings and experiences, many of which are shared by MSers.

Brecher, E. and the Editors of Consumer Reports: *Love, Sex, and Aging.* Boston, Little Brown, 1984. ($19.95)
Based on a survey of healthy aging people (50-90 years old). Contains information on sexual physiology. Many comments and ideas on how people cope with changing sexual function.

Comfort, A.: *The Joy of Sex.* New York, Simon and Schuster 1974 ($11.95).

Comfort, A.: *More Joy.* New York, Simon and Schuster, 1975. ($11.95)

Through text and drawings, these books explore a wide variety of sexual activities. They are oriented toward athletic sex with orgasm as the goal, but there are useful ideas. A book to enjoy with your partner.

Miles, H. J.: *Sexual Happiness in Marriage*. Grand Rapids, Zondervan Publishing House, 1967. (Available in Christian bookstores $3.95)
A marriage manual written from a Christian perspective. It has a good discussion of timing differences between men and women. This book is addressed primarily to young engaged couples. Its frank and reassuring message should prove helpful to others as well.

Mooney, T. O.; Cole, T. M.; Chilgren, R. A.: *Sexual Options for Paraplegics and Quadriplegics*. Boston, Little Brown, 1975. ($9.95)
Specifically directed toward people with spinal cord injuries. Contains explicit photographs. Geared to men more than women, but helpful for both.

Zilbergeld, B.: *Male Sexuality*. New York, Bantam, 1978. ($4.95)
An excellent book for men and women. Discusses myths about what male sex is supposed to be. Then offers specific suggestions for counteracting the myths and becoming aware of your real sexual needs. Gives many exercises for dealing with problems in achieving erection, ejaculatory control, and so on. The style is entertaining and serious. MSers will find the lack of pressure to perform particularly helpful.

REFERENCES:

1) American Association of Sex Educators, Counselors, and Therapists, 11 Du Pont Circle N.W., Suite 220, Washington, D.C., 20036.

2) Barbach, L.: *For Each Other*. New York, Signet, 1982. ($3.95)

3) Barbach, L.: *For Yourself: the Fulfillment of Female Sexuality*. New York, Signet, 1975.

4) Crisisline, National Gay Task Force. Call 1-(800) 221-7044, or 1-(212)-807-6016 in New York State, 3:00 to 9:00 P.M., E.S.T., Monday through Friday.

5) Eve's Garden, 119 W. 57th St., New York, NY, 10019.

6) Masters, W.; Johnson, V.: *Human Sexual Inadequacy*. Boston, Little Brown, 1970; p. 67.

7) Support Group, Lesbians/Gays with disabilities, P.O. Box 7445, Minneapolis, MN, 55407.

8) Valleroy, M.; Kraft, G.: Sexual Dysfunction in Multiple Sclerosis. *Arch. Phys. Med. Rehab.* Vol. 65, pages 125–128, 1984.

9) Xandria Collection, Lawrence Research Group, P.O. Box 31039, San Francisco, CA, 94131 (Ask for the free catalogue for the disabled.) Phone: 1-(415)-864-5406

10) Zilbergeld, B.: *Male Sexuality*. New York, Bantam, 1978.

Chapter 16

Managing the
Patient-Doctor Relationship
By John K. Wolf

The realization comes to me that we are equal.
I am not less because I am imperfect.
The stereotype is fiction, designed
By minds frightened of the unknown.

I have believed the fiction
Because I have known no different.
But I am being eaten alive by death.
And the part of me that's still alive, wants to live
Until it's time to die.

You and I must overcome the chains of fear.
Together we must write the new story.

Bonnie Johannes
September, 1985

PROFESSIONAL ASPECTS OF THE RELATIONSHIP

What do you expect to get from your doctor, and what do you expect to give? This patient-doctor relationship will last for many years, so it is to your advantage to answer that question now.

My answer? 1) Get precise information during each office visit about how this disease affects your body. 2) Discuss with the doctor your present concerns and needs. Think about them carefully beforehand, so your brief conversation can be useful to you when you leave. Efficient communication helps the doctor practice a better brand of medicine, and provides more thoughtful care for you. If you achieve these two goals, you will both understand each other better.

You have probably disagreed with us elsewhere in this volume. You may disagree with me even more as you read this chapter, because patients and doctors often have different goals. I shall discuss here some of the ideas your doctor may have, and some of the factors that interfere with the relationship. I hope this will help you understand your doctor's actions. Let us first examine doctors and modern doctoring.

Education of a Modern Medic

Medical students begin as idealists. They imagine themselves in the future as caring physicians, who will know every patient intimately and be able to respond immediately to any request. They plan to worry about each patient individually and perhaps to wait by the phone for a call. Naturally they will be completely informed about all areas of modern medical practice. They will have acquired the wisdom that comes with age before their 30th birthday.

Reality arrives when medical students face the pressures of training and the exhaustion of internship and residency. As practicing physicians mature, they encounter insoluble problems of diagnosis and management. Difficult cases consume time set aside for family and for sleep. The telephone jangles unwelcome news into an already overcrowded day and night. Chronic illness and chronic despair wrench at us from all directions. As modern physicians, we expect to be effective. When we are not, we wonder: could someone else have done better? There is no end to the need, but there is an end to energy, wakefulness, and even to compassion.

Eventually, successful physicians discover that they can only bleed from a few pores, and with a few people at one time. The rest must wait. We learn the limits of our knowledge and skill. We harden our hearts to what must happen to our patients, and go on. Those who fail to harden under the heat of practice, quit, or change to a less demanding field of medicine. Or they burn out. Or worse. The hardening process is necessary, but it takes its toll. Because of it, hardened physicians are often less lovely people.

We doctors are people, just like you. Our limits are similar to yours. We cannot give more than we have. We cannot do more than we know. We cannot practice medicine 24 hours a day and survive. If you understand these things, perhaps you can accept us for what we have become, and use us for what we do well.

Diagnosis and Management are Meat and Potatoes

Modern medical practice at its most elementary level demands accurate diagnosis, followed by effective suggestions for treatment. These are the only services a doctor can provide that no one else can. Consult other professionals or acquaintances for your other problems.

In times past, people hired a physician because he had a warm bedside manner, or because he lived nearby. In those times, there was little treatment for *any* illness, so the doctor's personality was paramount. His primary job was to provide comfort and ease pain. With the advent of effective treatment for specific diseases, amiability has become less important. Now, a missed diagnosis or failed therapy can mean the difference between recovery and death.

Everything Else is Gravy

Once diagnosis and management plans are established, many physicians recommend community services, such as the Visiting Nurses and physical therapy programs, the best place to buy a wheelchair, agencies or individuals for personal and family counseling. But as a practice becomes more demanding, busy doctors must concentrate on doing what they do best: diagnosis and treatment.

Choose Your Doctor with Care

Begin your search with a clear mind. Seek competence first, friendship second. Once you have found an able physician, be doubly happy if you also like each other. For help with your other needs, seek other specialists in the caring professions.

My editors were concerned with this section:

> "How can MSers trust a doctor's competence when they know MS cannot be diagnosed with certainty by anyone? What is effective treatment, when no one can cure me? I want to get well, but no doctor can do that for me!"

I do not have sure-fire answers to these questions. Look around. Ask at the local MS Society. Talk to other

MSers and friends. The real problem is to distinguish competence from amiability and a warm bedside manner. Choose competence above everything else.

Fractionation of Medical Care is a Necessity

MSers need neurologists to diagnose MS, and to teach them management of MS symptoms. When you have absorbed the contents of this primer on MS management and have learned everything your neurologist can teach you, you will earn your "PhD in MS Management." Then your neurologist will become less important to you, and symptoms of unrelated illness will demand attention the neurologist cannot give.

MSers have about the same chance as anyone else of catching a cold, developing cancer, or becoming pregnant. So MSers need primary care specialists, like internists and family practitioners, who are expert at diagnosis and management of symptoms unrelated to MS. Even with your PhD-MS, what do you know about pneumonia, anemia, heart trouble, stomach ulcers? What experience does your neurologist have with these diseases? A neurologist can refer you to an internist, family practitioner, or to an appropriate specialist, but do not expect a neurologist's expertise to extend much beyond the nervous system.

Fractionation of medical care makes life more uncertain. When a new symptom appears, you may not know whom to call. You can benefit from the complexity of medical care if you approach it with intelligence, not frightened helplessness. As different practitioners offer their expertise, your knowledge and understanding will increase. Once you have learned what each practitioner has to teach, choose management plans that best suit you.

Special Problems of Chronic Disease.

The problems of chronic disease are different from those of brief illnesses. Some physicians do well with acute illness and mild disability, but not with the more serious problems of advanced disease. Recognize the boundaries of your physician's expertise, and when necessary seek other sources of support. This way, both you and your physician will avoid feeling angry and hurt.

MSers pose a special problem for doctors. As we care for you, we begin to like you, individually, and as a group. You are generally young, pleasant people. Your children are almost as beautiful as our own. Soon, you become an important part of our professional family. Our secretaries know your voices on the phone, and often have personal relationships with you that are quite separate from our own. Because of this affection, it pains us when you get sick.

This is especially true of slowly progressing MS. After a few years of slowly progressing disability, doctor and patient relax. Each new symptom has gone away before. But there may come a time when the illness begins to accelerate.

As patient and physician face this new and frightening situation, the old easy friendship *must change*, because friendship and anxiety interfere with best medical judgement. Now, all the doctor's energy must be trained on the new problems. When you begin to call the office asking frantic questions, you probably know there are no answers, but you must ask. It is a cry for reassurance that can no longer be given.

Your doctor may no longer return your calls promptly. You may wait three days, and then find yourself speaking to the secretary, not the doctor. When you break down and weep on the phone, you may get prescriptions for Valium!

The doctor may even get upset on the phone and shout: "Well, you have MS, what do you expect me to *do!*" The hurt, anger and frustration at both ends of the line are palpable in that cry. The doctor hangs up shaken, ashamed and angry, angry at himself for behaving so badly, and at you for making him feel that way! You may be left weeping helplessly at home, cursing the physician, the disease and anyone else handy.

Doctor *and* patient need solace at this point. Your doctor may be able to phone or write to set things straight. If that happens, accept the olive branch. Both of you need it.

If he cannot, you have several options. You can sit home helpless, with new symptoms you do not understand. You can change doctors. Or, if you know that your doctor has your best interests at heart, even if he was overwhelmed today, you can get to work and help *him.* Doctoring and patienting is a two-way street, and just now he needs your help as much as you need his. Swallow your hurt and anger. Write to him.

"Dear Dr.

What a terrible set-to we had today (yesterday, last week). I realize this disease of mine is at fault. I heard the frustration and anger in your voice, and I know you are as helpless as I am.

Please. May I come in to talk with you? I want no miracle. I do need advice about my bladder, and I want to know whether the new symptom I mentioned to you on the phone is caused by my MS or by some other thing.

I may cry when we meet as I did on the phone. Pay no attention when I do it, it's just my way. I *hate* this disease. I want to continue to work with you to fight it as we have done in the past. Please have your secretary call to say when I may come in.

Best regards,

It may not work. Some physicians cannot take care of patients with advancing disease. Some of us back away and move on to other problems. Some of us have set-to's on the phone because things are going badly at home, or because of the pressures of other sick patients in the practice. Like you, physicians are limited people, with limited tolerance.

If you cannot patch things up, find another physician who can cope with more advanced MS. Let the new doctor know from the start that yours is a more complex case. On your first visit, tell your new doctor you know that doctoring has limitations, but you need help within those limits.

"We'll do our best together."

If you have advanced MS, consider relying on an internist or family practitioner. Years of experience have taught you more than enough about aids to ambulation and management of spasticity. You can learn catheter care from an internist as easily as from a neurologist. Hospital care for pneumonia or bladder infection may be even better on a medical service. Preventive inoculation against pneumonia is part of the yearly autumn practice of many internists and family practitioners, not of most neurologists. Think it over. As you change doctors, you may also decide to change specialties.

In small communities there is little choice of doctors. If this is the case, use your physician for the things he knows best, and other people for their special knowledge. This will relieve the strain on both you and your doctor. Tell your doctor what you are doing to help yourself, and use his competence in the practice of medicine.

Violent Dissent Accepted

I showed this chapter to a bright medical student, Dr. Chris Butler. He commented strongly:

"It is not unreasonable for patients to expect warmth, honesty and sympathy from other human beings. I do not expect a doctor to be a superior human being, but I do expect a doctor to be human, at the very *least.*

"*You* excuse doctors who are unwilling or unable to offer proper emotional support to their patients. You have not convinced *me* that just because we have more diagnostic and therapeutic options, we should be allowed to sell our patients short emotionally. Even if other people can offer comfort, and only doctors can make a diagnosis, that is no reason for doctors to abdicate their responsibility to give emotional support.

"You state that a modern physician must before everything else be an accurate diagnostician. Agreed, but without interpersonal skills, the physician is also useless. The uncaring doctor cannot take a first-rate history, nor perform as thorough an examination. These are still the most important parts of the diagnostic process. Surely confidence and trust materially affect the course of recovery. In any case, isn't a patient's comfort in a disease like MS one of the most important things a doctor should be thinking about?"

He's right, of course. I do not mean to excuse doctors for our failings. Unfortunately, most people have a limited choice of doctors. None of us is perfect. We all have times of *great* failure, when we need your help as much as you have needed ours. But you can still profit from an imperfect relationship. Like Chris Butler, I know MSers consider it important for them and their doctors to like and understand each other. You will find it easier to follow advice from a physician you like and trust, than from one you find offensive.

Make your choice from a list of competent physicians in your community. If one of these doctors has a warm bedside manner and a genuine interest in you as a person, that would be excellent. But beware the physician whose only asset is his bedside manner. That person belongs in Chapter 20!

One Last Word About Doctors

Most physicians are pleased that we became doctors, but the practice of medicine consumes physicians. We marry and raise children as other people do. We, too, need to relax on days off, and to have quiet times at home. Office and hospital hours are never long enough to accomplish the tasks at hand. Remember. Every minute spent in extra conversation with you must be stolen from someone else, or stolen from the family or from sleep.

Physicians are not superhuman. We have no extraordinary powers of understanding, observation or compassion. Your doctor is probably not the most intelligent person you have ever met, nor the best informed. We become depressed, divorced, alcoholic and burned out just as other people do. The special skills we have learned are valuable to some people. But they are all that sets us apart from anyone else.

You may call on a Thursday and learn that this is doctor's afternoon off. Instead of sneering at such an easy life, remember why you had to wait three hours in the E.R. one Sunday morning. Although the doctor had been in the hospital long before you arrived, he had to finish ward rounds before he could attend to you. Doctoring is a busy business. If they do it well, your doctors earn their keep.

Do not look *up* to your doctor. Look *at* your doctor. Discuss *together* issues you can handle well together. Ask where to look for information about other problems, but do not expect infallibility. Above all, do not relinquish to your doctor or to anyone else the major decisions that govern your life.

MS is only one part of your life and your doctor plays a small role in its management. If you approach your physician with this attitude, you will both feel better about your relationship in the long run. Together you can laugh occasionally, cry when necessary. The main thing is to depend on each other in your fight against this disease.

LANGUAGE *VERSUS* COMMUNICATION

Imprecise language causes problems of communication between MSers and their doctors:

The MSer:

"Why is it so hard to tell a doctor about my symptoms? They see so many people, why don't they understand? Why do doctors so often get my history wrong after I have been so careful to tell them everything I know? Don't they even care? What's *wrong* with them?"

The Doctor:

"Why is it so hard for patients to say simply and directly what has happened to them? Don't they live all day long with their symptoms? Don't they think about their symptoms? Why can't they simply *spit it out?* What's *wrong* with people who can't tell such a simple thing as their own history without total confusion?"

The trouble is with the words. Take a baby-simple word like "numbness," for example. You speak of a "numb" tooth, meaning a tooth injected with an anesthetic. You speak of a "numb leg," meaning paralysis; a "numb arm" meaning incoordination. If you tell your physician that your legs are "numb," and mean spasticity has made it hard to walk, how is the doctor to know? If an MSer says he fell, a doctor, having fallen, understands. If an MSer describes the numbness of local anesthesia, the doctor comprehends, having had a similar experience.

But what term describes your perception of spasticity in the legs? What word communicates the sensation caused by an MS plaque in the spinal cord, that damages —partially—one of the sensory pathways? Perhaps not even another *MSer* has had that precise sensation, so there is no word for it.

Words originate in the everyday experience of the people who use them. Special words transmit highly complex and precise information between two astronomers discussing an observation in the heavens. Household words transmit accurate information about daily events. The MSer is stuck with this language, which is inadequate to describe MS.

To cope with the problem of faulty communication between doctor and patient, most medical schools offer courses to teach skills in medical history taking. Although this is an inadequate solution, it is a start.

Next time you visit your physician, note how your language affects the understanding you and your doctor have of your illness. Note how the physician's language promotes or detracts from your comprehension of the options you have for management. You will find that many problems between you are not due to personality, but to linguistic misunderstandings.

In the end, MSers skilled in management techniques can often help each other more than we can help from the outside. Among MSers there is a commonality of experience and therefore of language that we physicians can never share. Last, MSers spend more time with each other than they do with their doctors, so they have a better chance to understand each other. Learn everything you can about your own illness and its management. Then you and fellow MSers can share and teach one another better management for a better life.

"It's Not Just the Patient Who Speaks a Foreign Language!"

—Said Bernice and Mike, when they read this. "What about the problems that result when doctors talk jargon?" Doctors use technical terms because they are precise, and because they are used to them. Doctors don't remember that patients can't understand them.

"For fear of looking stupid, patients may be reluctant to ask the meaning when they don't understand the doctor. You had better mention this problem, or a lot of readers will be angry that you have discussed only the patient's use of language! Tell people to *ask* what's meant when they're not sure!"

Sorry about that, readers. This book is full of recommendations that you take charge. Take charge of your body. Learn about your medications. Take charge of relationships with your family, your friends, your work and your doctor. When we speak Greek, stop us!

Write it Down

Now that you have begun to understand how language interferes with communication, remember your goal: to give and receive as much information as possible during the brief time you spend with your physician. It serves your purpose to be efficient.

Ask your doctor if a letter would be useful before each office visit. If the answer is "no," make a list so you will remember all your questions.

A letter can provide a very efficient beginning to conversation. Usually I glance at such a letter before the office visit, but I do not study it. The letter serves as a guide to conversation in the office, not as a detailed communication. It channels our energies toward the patient's concerns as we talk.

Type your letter if you can. Make it short and concise. Think of it as an agenda for discussion.

"Dear Dr. Wolf,

I am coming to see you on Thursday because two weeks ago my right thumb went numb. Now I can't use the hand. Is there anything we can do about it?

I also am having trouble with my bladder and need to talk bladder management with you.

Best regards,"

Often people list five to ten individual concerns, each expressed *briefly* in the note. If you do this, you and your doctor will be sure to discuss them all.

Try Paul Cohen's Flowsheet!

As my friend and colleague, Paul Cohen, read this text before publication, he devised a brief chart* for use by patient and doctor during their discussions. Section I contains basic information for the inside cover of your chart, at home or at the office. Section II may help you through the office discussion without forgetting important issues.

Fill out Section I as you progress through your MS, keeping important dates and figures instantly available. Between visits, keep a copy of section II posted on the refrigerator, so you can jot things down as they occur to

---

* Note: The Flowsheet for MSers may be found on page 295-297.

you. Then write ahead if your doctor likes notes, or bring it with you.

TWO IMPORTANT HINTS FOR GETTING INFORMATION

1) The office telephone rings incessantly. Unless there are defined phoning hours, it interferes with the secretary's work and interrupts the doctor's concentration on other patients. If a call must be returned later, it takes that much more time for everyone, including the patient. So what is the best way to ask a routine question, unrelated to an emergency? By mail.

Physicians set aside time for letters. Some, like myself, type our answers, even if we make errors. Others like to scribble a reply on your note and send it back to you. If you have a series of questions, and your doctor likes to scribble, leave spaces for the replies between questions. Ask your doctor which is best.

Answers to letters are usually better thought out than answers on the phone in the midst of a hectic day. You can re-read a letter with a complex answer, but can you trust your memory of a phone conversation?

2) Where can you find the best information about the management of MS? In the community of MSers, of course. Use your local MS Society Chapter to meet other MSers. Ask senior MSers, who have been there and know. Provide information to junior MSers who still are learning. Spread useful information as far as you can. Where do you think nearly every page of this book originated?

You can contribute by writing to us, as other people have. Together, we can improve this volume to live up to its name. We cannot do it without your help.

Flowsheet for MSers
By
Paul S. Cohen, M.D.

Section I. Chart Face Sheet Data

DIAGNOSTICS:
1) Date of first MS symptom: _____
2) Date of clinically definite diagnosis of MS _____
3) Dates of CT or MRI scans, and results:

_____   _____

_____   _____

4) Visual Evoked Potentials.
   Date _____ Result: Left _____ Right _____
5) Auditory Evoked Potentials.
   Date _____ Result _____
6) Cystometrogram.
   Date _____ Result _____
7) Lumbar Puncture.
   Date _____

Protein, Sugar? _____   Oligoclonal Bands? _____
Gamma globulin? _____   Myelin Basic Protein? ___

MANAGEMENT TECHNIQUES:

Aids to Ambulation?
Cane _____   Ankle splint _____

(Canadian) Crutches _____   Manual Wheelchair _____

Walker _____   Electric Wheelchair _____

Physical care:
Home nurse _____   Phone _____
Physical Therapist _____   Phone _____
Personal or family counselor _____   Phone _____

Medications:
Current medications, dates
Best dose, Lioresal _____ Date_____
Best dose, antidepressant _____ Date _____
Other medications, dose, date

_____   _____
_____   _____
_____   _____
_____   _____

ACTH or Prednisone. Dates, result of treatment.

_____   _____
_____   _____
_____   _____
_____   _____

Section II. MSer Office Visit Checklist

I need to discuss these unresolved issues with the doctor during the next visit, so we can make management decisions.

Major Purpose of the Visit: _____

Other Issues to Discuss

Mobility problems
Aids to mobility
Am I in an exacerbation?
Visual problems
  Double vision
  Loss of vision
Muscle weakness
Muscle spasms
Tremor
Incoordination

Laboratory Results
Depression
Insomnia?
Anxiety?
Bowels and Bladder
Sexual function
Pain
Physical therapy
Medications

_____
_____

Non-MS problems that require attention:

_____

_____

Management problems recently solved, which might be
useful for the next patient:

_____

_____

Section Four

Medical aspects:

Anatomy,
Diagnosis,
Prognosis,
Quackery,
Research

Introduction

We have discussed the art of living despite disability. In this section, you will find information about brain and spinal cord anatomy, which may help you to understand why your symptoms occur as they do.

We discuss the process of diagnosis. "How do I *know* my diagnosis of MS is accurate?" You don't. But if you have traveled with a careful clinician, you have less than a one percent chance that your diagnosis of MS was wrong.

"How much disability will I have ten years from now?" Much of the answer to this question depends on you. Have you adopted consistent and excellent bladder management techniques? Then your bladder will not be scarred and infected ten years from now. Are you inventive in your response to each aspect of disability? Are you *determined* to pursue mobility, regardless? Then despite disability you will be active. But just now, there is nothing any of us can do to prevent the accumulation of MS plaques in your brain and spinal cord.

You *can* predict the course of that part of your MS with some accuracy. You can define the limits of prediction. Then you can make realistic plans, based on that knowledge.

Quackery plagues MSers. Readers know there is still no cure. Readers know that no medication, no treatment changes the ultimate course of MS. Yet MSers search for the next possible treatment with tenacity unmatched by other groups of neurological patients. As you search, vultures wait to exploit your hopes and take your money. When this book appears in print, several new treatment fads will have appeared. Beware the fads. Judge the clinicians who offer them. Clear your mind of hope, so you can decide each time, whether this one finally is the cure, or only the most recent false hope.

Chapter 17

Anatomy and Function of the Nervous System for MSers
By John K. Wolf

INTRODUCTION

We cannot hope to understand the nervous system completely, but we know enough about its structure and function to understand many symptoms of MS. As you read this chapter, think about anatomy and function in terms of your own experience with MS.

ANATOMY OF NERVE CELLS (Neurons)

Neurons are built to carry messages for short or long distances in the body. Some are confined to the brain and spinal cord in the *central* nervous system. Others live in other body tissues, outside the central nervous system. These form the *peripheral* nervous system. All neurons have three major parts: the dendritic zone, the cell body and one axon (Fig. 17-1).

The Dendritic Zone
There are as many as 80,000 receptive sites on the dendritic zone of a single neuron. Each site receives messages from another neuron that may be far distant in

the nervous system. Some of those neurons transmit inhibitory messages that tend to stop the receiver from firing. Others transmit excitatory messages that tend to activate the receiving neuron. The dendritic tree accumulates all the excitatory and inhibitory impulses and sends a coordinated message down to the cell body: "Fire once!" or "Fire a whole volley!" or "*Stop!*"

The Dendritic zone of a neuron is usually thinner than other parts of the neuron and has no myelin covering. These two characteristics slow the conduction of impulses along this portion of the neuron, resulting in a prolonged alteration of electrical charge after a message arrives. This is the most elemental method used by the nervous system to handle the passage of time, and represents the simplest form of memory for recent events. Impulses reaching the dendritic zone are "remembered" as an altered membrane charge for a few milliseconds, a few minutes or even for a few hours. This alteration of electrical charge affects the firing pattern of that nerve cell while it lasts.

Cell Body

All cellular activity is ultimately controlled from the nucleus, illustrated inside the cell body in Figure 17-1. The nucleus contains the genes, which are the basic chemical determinant of life.

The portion of the cell body outside the nucleus is the factory where chemical reactions produce energy needed to run the cell and manufacture proteins, carbohydrates and fats. Cell membranes and the sub-cellular organs are formed in the cell body from these raw materials throughout its lifetime. There is no replacement for worn out nerve cells, so the process of cellular

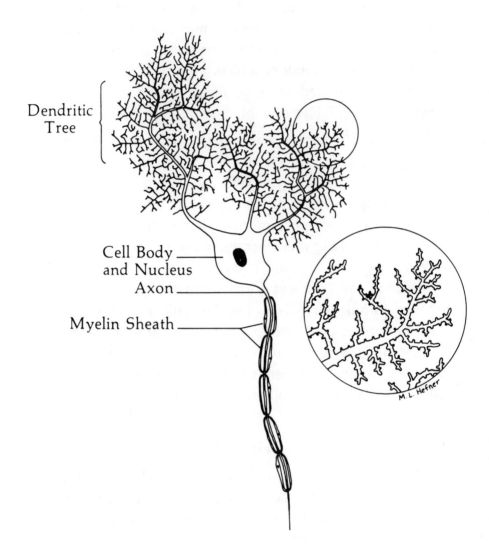

Dendritic
Tree

Cell Body
and Nucleus
Axon

Myelin Sheath

M. L. Hefner

Fig. 17-1. Drawing of a neuron emphasizes the large number of dendritic spines. Each spine accepts information from the axon of another neuron. The myelin sheath is made of individual myelin-forming cells that surround the axon with their bodies.

maintenance and repair is of great importance in the nervous system.

Axon

Axons are unthinking wires that transmit neuronal messages. Each axon terminal connects to one or more receptive sites on the dendritic zone of the next neuron or to the receptive site on a muscle or a gland.

The largest axons are covered by fatty insulation called myelin, which promotes rapid conduction down the axon. The large diameter allows an increased flow of electrical charge, just as a larger wire conducts more electricity in your home. Thus, large, myelinated axons transmit precise information rapidly across great distances in the nervous system.

Smaller unmyelinated axons, and axons with intermediate amounts of myelin have their own normal but slower conduction velocity. Short axons innervate neurons in the immediate neighborhood. Activity in chains of small neurons provides for the general background of body sensation and posture, and provides the complexity of human thought in the cortex of the brain.

Myelin

Myelin is the fatty coating that covers many axons in the central and peripheral nervous system. Special cells form myelin by wrapping themselves tightly around axons, insulating them from outside influences with their bodies. Unlike the insulation around telephone wires, myelin is a living substance that may be damaged by disease. Some diseases damage myelin-forming cells in the peripheral nervous system only. Others, like MS, damage myelin-forming cells only in the central nervous system.

305

If myelin is damaged, we say the axon is *demyelinated*. Transmission is slowed as a message passes through the demyelinated segment of axon, so the message arrives late, or not at all. Late arrival of one part of the total message from the brain can result in a poorly coordinated response, or no response at all.

Symptoms of MS result from globular regions of demyelination in the brain and spinal cord, called plaques. MS plaques interrupt messages traveling through the region. MS symptoms are the result: Slowed movements, uncoordinated movements, loss of feeling, loss of control.

SENSORY PATHWAYS IN THE BRAIN AND SPINAL CORD

Only three sensory tracts are available for direct examination; *pain* and *position sense* from the body, and *vision*. They carry specific messages, so neurologists may use them in diagnosis.

Pain Perception from the Body

Perception of pinprick is illustrated in Figure 17-2. The message is shown traveling in the thinner dark blue line to the spinal cord from the fingertip. Close inspection of the figure reveals a second neuron immediately inside the spinal cord (arrow) that picks up the initial discharge, crosses to the opposite side of the spinal cord and disappears from the figure as it turns upward toward the brain in the bundle called the lateral spinothalamic tract. Damage to this bundle causes loss of pinprick sensation on the body below the lesion. Notice that pinprick perception is lost on the *opposite* side of the body from the lesion, because the fibers cross

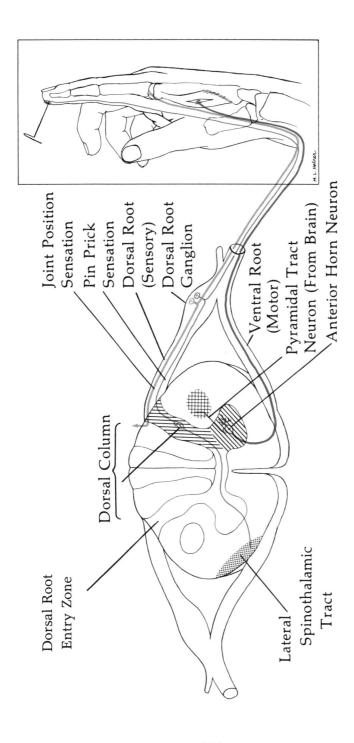

Joint Position
Sensation

Pin Prick
Sensation

Dorsal Root
(Sensory)

Dorsal Root
Ganglion

Ventral Root
(Motor)

Pyramidal Tract
Neuron (From Brain)

Anterior Horn Neuron

Dorsal Column

Dorsal Root
Entry Zone

Lateral
Spinothalamic
Tract

Fig. 17-2. The sensory pathways. See text for discussion.

the midline to reach the lateral spinothalamic tract before they ascend the spinal cord. Damage at this level causes loss of pain perception from the entire opposite side of the body below the level of the damage, because lower segments have already contributed their fibers to the tract.

Most MSers have experienced "numbness from here on down," and were then unable to feel a pinprick in the numb area. If you have such a "sensory level" now, test yourself with a common pin and discover the exact borders of the sensory change. Now you know that the numbness is caused by damage to the lateral spinothalamic tract on the opposite side of the spinal cord at the level where pinprick returns to normal. By knowing this one small piece of neuroanatomy you have located one MS plaque precisely. During the rest of a neurological examination, other precisely localized areas of sensory or motor dysfunction can demonstrate the presence of more than one discrete lesion in the white matter of the central nervous system—a point of great importance as we shall see in the next chapter.

The Body's Sense of Position and Movement

Look again at the woman's right hand in Fig. 17-2. The thicker, light blue nerve fiber carries information about the motion and position of her finger at any particular moment. This fiber travels up the arm and enters the spinal cord, accompanied by similar nerve fibers from other joints and the skin.

Is the finger bent? How much? Is it moving? In what direction? How fast? Like the lateral spinothalamic tract, this thicker fiber carries precise information rapidly in a "private line" from the finger of her right hand to the parietal cortex on the left side of her brain. Note that this fiber enters the dorsal column bundles *without* crossing to the opposite side of the spinal cord and without a connection to another neuron. Damage to the posterior column in the spinal cord causes loss of position and movement sense below the lesion, but on the *same side* of the body as the damage.

When the posterior column axon reaches the medulla in the brainstem (Fig. 17-3), there is a connection to the second neuron. The second neuron refines the message and sends its axon to the opposite side of the brainstem and courses to the brain.

Symptoms of posterior column damage are common among MSers but the symptoms are usually harder to recognize than loss of pain perception. Sometimes an MSer cannot tell what is in a pocket. Legs may not walk properly unless the MSer looks where the feet are going. Usually the complaint is clumsiness, sometimes "numbness" or "puffiness." MSers have a hard time finding the proper word for this sensory symptom, and this results in some of the linguistic problems we discussed on pages 290–293.

To test position sense, close your eyes, while someone moves your great toe or a small joint in one finger. Normally, people can detect a millimeter or two of movement in a great toe, and even smaller movements in the small joints of the fingers. If you sense that a hand or a leg malfunctions, and you cannot feel movements of the joints, there is probably a lesion in the posterior column on the same side of the spinal cord. Discovering the *level* of position sense loss is more difficult than finding the level of pinprick loss. You probably will need help from a neurologist to determine precisely the location of the lesion.

These two sensory tracts of the central nervous sys-

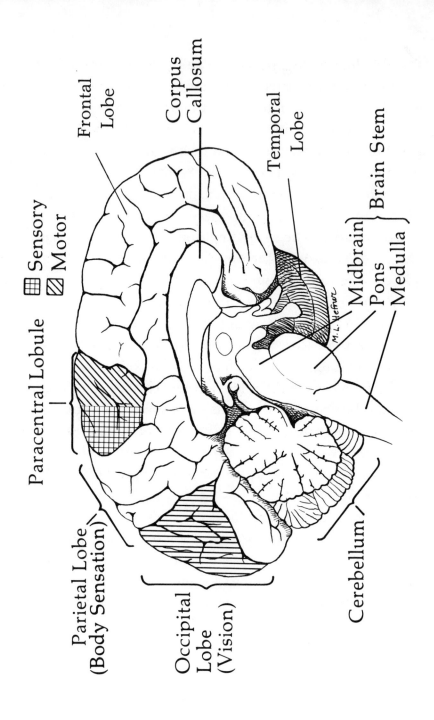

Fig. 17-3. Gross anatomy of the brain. Anatomical landmarks are mentioned in the text.

310

tem are of great value in diagnosis. An examiner can determine the level ("from here on down") of one or more lesions, on either the *left* or the *right* side of the *anterior* (loss of pain sense) or the *posterior* (loss of position sense) part of the spinal cord, using only a pin for equipment, and fingers to wiggle joints or skin.

Vision

Most MSers have experienced at least temporary loss of vision. Like the pathways for body sensation, visual impulses travel in tightly packed bundles that carry the most detailed information the nervous system ever receives. About 90% of optic nerve axons serve the few degrees of central vision where detailed visual discrimination occurs.

An MS plaque in the optic nerve usually causes loss of visual acuity or blindness. The complaint is blurred vision, inability to read fine print or an actual blind spot in the central field of vision of one eye (a central scotoma). This is often accompanied by pain when moving the eye. The diagnosis is optic neuritis, or retrobulbar neuritis. (See also page 159.)

MS plaques rarely destroy the entire nerve, so visual acuity can return to normal or nearly normal when inflammation and swelling subside. Undamaged optic nerve fibers also come from that central portion of the retina and serve visual acuity as best they can. If enough are damaged, there is permanent diminution of visual acuity, because there are not enough remaining fibers. Most MSers retain visual acuity of 20/70 or better. The text in this volume is set so that a person with 20/70 visual acuity can read it.

Friends and family often ask MSers why they don't just get glasses to correct visual loss, as other people do.

Glasses help to focus light on the retina of the eye, so the image is sharper. But if nerve cells that serve the retina are damaged, no amount of focusing improves the image.

The forward end of the optic nerve, called the *optic nerve head,* is visible through the ophthalmoscope. Normally the nerve head is pink or orange in color and has many tiny blood vessels on its surface. After an attack of optic neuritis the nerve head becomes pale as it loses some of those blood vessels and myelin. This pale appearance is called *optic atrophy,* a common finding among MSers. Even without visible optic atrophy, an electronic test, called *visual evoked responses,* can reveal evidence of demyelination. How? By demonstrating slowed nerve impulse conduction through demyelinated visual pathways. Visual evoked responses are discussed more fully on pages 343–344.

Sensory Integration in the Parietal Lobes

In the sensory system alone there are about a million fibers passing through the upper spinal cord. They are on their way to many parts of the brainstem and brain. The mixture of active nerve fibers varies, depending on the person's moment-to-moment activity. An increase in the firing frequency of any single neuron, or in the number of neurons firing transmits urgency. The total firing pattern determines not only the location, but also the quality of the information; so that we distinguish a pinprick from a bee sting, a loving touch from a slap.

All sensory messages from the right hand travel to the same part of the left parietal cortex. There they are correlated with similar information arriving in adjacent parts of the cortex. Information flowing from that piece of cortex moves directly to motor areas that control the same hand and finger, as well as to other parts of the brain.

The sensory cortex of the brain receives visual information in the occipital lobes, hearing in the temporal lobes and bodily sensation in the parietal lobes. (See Fig. 17-3.) These raw sensations are processed, evaluated and stored (remembered!) over large areas of the cerebral cortex. Motor pathways from the brain permit it to express its decision to *do* something in response to the outside world.

MOTOR PATHWAYS IN THE BRAIN AND SPINAL CORD

Pyramidal Tract

An important motor bundle originates in the cortex of the frontal lobe. It communicates directly with motor neurons in the anterior horns of the spinal cord to activate fine motor control: tying shoelaces, buttoning buttons or writing. This bundle, which forms a small part of the pyramidal tract, is called the corticospinal tract. It is illustrated in Fig. 17-2 as a red fiber leaving the tight bundle on the lateral part of the spinal cord and going to the anterior horn neuron.

Before reaching the spinal cord neurons, the corticospinal tract has been joined by axons from many other parts of the brain. Together, they orchestrate the motor response. This entire bundle is now called the pyramidal tract. The "orchestra" within the pyramidal tract helps to specify body posture at all levels of the spinal cord and adjusts muscle tone to adapt to changing centers of gravity. Related motor systems move the head and eyes so the brain can observe the results of its work. While the bulk of the pyramidal tract provides

313

this background, the corticospinal tract directs the specific act. It is the piccolo, carrying a melody of personal response against the background of the whole orchestra. We listen to the piccolo, so we think of *it* as the response, but without the background orchestration, the melody would fall flat.

Symptoms of pyramidal tract disease include muscle tightness, ankle clonus, flexor spasms that jerk the leg spontaneously, exhaustion, loss of muscle power and paralysis.

Signs of Pyramidal tract disease include increased deep tendon reflexes such as the knee and elbow jerks, loss of muscle power and the presence of a superficial reflex called the Babinski sign. If Babinski's sign is present when the sole of the foot is scratched, the great toe moves up toward the head instead of down. This means there is a lesion in the pyramidal system that serves that leg. These symptoms and signs represent spasticity. Excellent treatment for some symptoms of spasticity is discussed in Chapter 4.

Anterior Horn Cells

Skeletal muscles receive their commands from anterior horn neurons in the spinal cord (Fig. 17-2). They perform the quick or repetitive movements our bodies need to stay alive in this dangerous world. Anterior horn neurons are the final target of all neuronal activity because of their direct command of skeletal muscles. Therefore, demyelination anywhere in the central nervous system *must* affect their function. Has something happened to your gait? Are your fingers incoordinated? If so, the anterior horn neurons in your spinal cord are getting garbled messages from the rest of your central nervous system.

Double Vision and the MLF

Medial longitudinal fasciculus (MLF): the very name frightens medical students. Actually, there is little mystery to the MLF. It is a small tract in the brainstem that coordinates movements of the eyes when they look left and right. When looking to the right, the left MLF turns the left eye to the right. When looking to the left, the right MLF turns the right eye to the left. Is that crystal clear now? No wonder medical students fear the MLF!

The MLF passes through a region of the brainstem that often accumulates MS plaques. These plaques are the usual cause of double vision among MSers. A plaque in the MLF interrupts coordinated movements of the eyeballs, so that they do not turn precisely together. This causes the MSer to receive two images instead of one.

The double vision may disappear or lessen after an attack, but a neurologist may detect minimal incoordination of eye movements with a simple examination. When the MSer looks rapidly to left and right, the eye that turns toward the nose may lag behind the one turning away. This picture tells the neurologist there has been damage to the MLF (1).*

Cerebellum

Unlike the pyramidal tract and the MLF, cerebellar connections have no direct effect on individual movements. Consequently cerebellar disease is discernible only as complex motor dysfunction. Damage to the cerebellum (Fig. 17-3) causes imbalance, and changes the speed and cadence of speech. Cerebellar incoordi-

* Note: The reference for this chapter may be found on page 325.

nation of willed movement resembles tremor. Abnormalities of eye movement occur after cerebellar damage. Each of these symptoms is disabling to a degree, but locating the plaques is more difficult than locating the lesions in sensory systems. Even so, when imbalance or tremor "looks cerebellar" to an experienced examiner, the cerebellum is usually involved.

Cerebellar activity never enters consciousness, so the MSer cannot clearly state why a hand misses or a leg walks wrong. Unlike other motor systems, the defect cannot be bypassed or improved through physical therapy. The cerebellum is a creature of the present. It has no ability to learn, so it continues to malfunction while other parts of the brain respond to accumulated experiences.

AUTONOMIC NERVOUS SYSTEM

The autonomic nervous system functions in parallel to the voluntary nervous system. It governs primitive functions like heart beat, blood pressure, hunger, sweating, bowel and bladder activity. It controls glands throughout the body. The autonomic nervous system is responsible for the developments that occur at puberty, and for continuing normal sexual function. It remains a world apart within our complex bodies, automatically doing basic functions that maintain life.

Autonomic functions are direct responses to commands that originate at a level of the spinal cord or brainstem. Most are completely uncontrollable by any act of will, for example:

> "Blood pressure, go to 120/70."
> "Constrict the pupil of the left eye."
> "Hunger!"

316

"Sweat!"

Ridiculous. People don't do that.

Some autonomic functions can be brought under momentary, but not complete control:

"Hold your breath."
"Urinate."
"Defecate."

If you hold your breath until you pass out, normal breathing resumes immediately. Have you tried to urinate or defecate when the laboratory wanted a sample? Impossible, unless your bladder or rectum was ready.

Some autonomic functions accompany willed or conscious activities, but they occur, or *fail* to occur, involuntarily. Sexual arousal comes from the brain, but male erection and ejaculation, and female vaginal lubrication and orgasm depend for their full expression on intact function of the autonomic nervous system. Fear also begins in the brain, but the increased heart and breathing rates, and the rise in blood pressure are involuntary.

The autonomic nervous system becomes important to MSers because of bowel, bladder and sexual dysfunction. MS plaques in the pyramidal tract, in the lowest portion of the spinal cord or in some sensory pathways, cause impairment of bowel and bladder control and loss of some sexual functions.

Anatomy of Bladder Malfunction

Two major kinds of bladder dysfunction plague MSers: spasticity and flaccidity. Usually, the MS bladder is a combination of both. Some MSers have even more complex malfunction of bladder and bladder neck muscles. Fortunately, there are effective management tech-

317

niques for all types of dysfunction. This section will be especially useful if you wish to understand more about the neural control of the bladder. Read it in conjunction with Chapter 5.

Spastic Bladder

When the normal bladder has filled, it does not empty without a direct command from the *person* living upstairs. Nerve fibers for bladder control travel down the spinal cord near the pyramidal tract (See pages 313–314.), whose fibers control arms and legs. Bladder spasticity usually results from MS plaques in and around the pyramidal tracts.

Spastic leg muscles contract too strongly when stretched. Hyperactive reflexes, clonus and spontaneous spasms result. Likewise, a spastic bladder develops spontaneous spasms when only partially filled. These cause sudden urgency and embarrassing incontinence. A purely spastic bladder is tight and contracted. When it has accumulated only an ounce or so of urine, it goes into uncontrolled spasms, so it can never fill completely.

Flaccid Bladder

Bladder flaccidity is the consequence of either or both of two distinctly different processes. When there is damage to the *motor centers* that supply muscles of the bladder wall, the muscles receive no *commands*. When there is damage to *sensory pathways* from the bladder, the brain and spinal cord receive no *information* about the fullness of the bladder, and no *stimulus* for voiding. In either case, the bladder changes from an active contractile organ that monitors and controls its volume, to a tired old bag that does not empty.

The MS Bladder

Bladder malfunction in MSers results from the combined effects of MS plaques at all levels of the central nervous system. Some cause bladder spasticity by interrupting higher pathways for bladder control. Some cause bladder flaccidity by interrupting pathways for bladder sensation or by damaging the sacral spinal cord. The balance between spastic *vs.* flaccid varies, as the number, placement and severity of MS plaques change during the MSer's lifetime.

MS bladders usually go into spasm after collecting only a small amount of urine. After the initial spasm there is less contractility, so the bladder fails to empty completely. Within the hour, a small amount of urine has again collected, renewing the spasms and the urgency.

This combination of spastic and flaccid bladder wall function may be further complicated by abnormalities of bladder neck muscles. MSers often have tremendous spasms of urgency but find they cannot urinate! Bladder neck muscles have gone into spasm simultaneously with the bladder wall. This is called detrusor-sphincter dyssynergia. (See page 121.)

At other times bladder neck muscles relax spontaneously, causing sudden incontinence, with or without urgency. If this happens to you, consider following a regular schedule of self-cath to keep the bladder from filling completely. You might also wear adult diapers or condom drainage and a leg bag, to control the incontinence that does occur.

Cystometrogram (Urodynamic Evaluation)

Many MSers can tell that bladder function is primarily flaccid. They have learned that Credé (See page

106.) helps to express more urine. Recurrent bladder infections and catheterization have proved to them that it empties incompletely. Other MSers know their bladder is primarily spastic. Why? Because they have significant spasticity in the legs and severe bladder spasms without evident bladder enlargement.

If the diagnosis is unclear, I recommend a cystometrogram. ("Cysto" means bladder. "Metro" means measurement. "Gram" means recording.) A cystometrogram measures and records bladder contractions as the bladder is filled. The procedure is simple. First, the patient voids and a catheter is placed in the bladder. The amount of urine remaining in the bladder is the residual urine volume. This figure determines many bladder management decisions. (See page 99.)

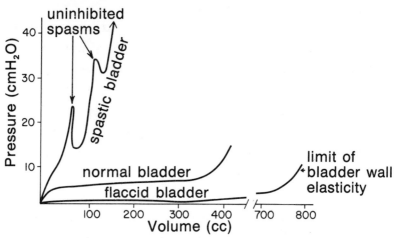

Fig. 17-4. Pressure-volume curves from cystometrograms. The text describes results of cystometric examinations for spastic, flaccid, and MS bladders.

Next, water or carbon dioxide gas is injected through the catheter into the bladder at a slow, even rate. Bladder pressure is recorded as the examination proceeds. These pressure-volume figures are the graphic display of the cystometrogram. If the bladder is normal (See Fig. 17-4.), the pressure rises immediately to about five to ten cm. of water (four to seven mm. Hg). As it fills, the normal bladder wall adjusts to the increasing volume with a gradual increase in pressure.

At a volume of 125 to 175 cc. (four to six ounces) and pressure of 10–15 cm water, normal bladders transmit the sensation of *first desire to void*. This can be suppressed voluntarily. Sensation of *Fullness* appears at 200 to 300 cc. (seven to ten ounces). Normally at a volume of 300 to 400 cc., there is a rapid rise in pressure as the bladder reaches its limit of elastic stretch. Increasing *urgency* is followed by *pain* at pressures of 30–35 cm. water. During a normal cystometrogram, normal fluctuations in bladder wall tone produce small pressure waves, but no uninhibited spasms.

A purely spastic bladder has almost no residual urine volume. At the very onset of bladder filling, the pressure rises to abnormally high levels. Soon, uninhibited spasms raise the pressure to 40–60 cm. water and hold it there. If pain pathways are intact, the spasms are agonizingly painful and the procedure is instantly stopped.

A large residual urine volume signals bladder flaccidity. Once the bladder has fully drained and the procedure begins, there is neither a steady rise in pressure, nor spontaneous pressure waves. Indeed, there is no pressure at all, until the bladder has filled almost to capacity. At that volume, the pressure rises rapidly, because the bladder wall can stretch no further.

The pressure-volume curve describes the *motor* side of bladder function. The patient describes the *sensory* side. The normal sensory pathways report a desire to void, a sense of fullness, urgency and pain at well defined pressure ranges. If in addition to severe spasticity a person has significant loss of sensation, a strong uninhibited spasm may cause only slight urgency. The same pressure in a person with normal sensation would cause severe pain.

Cystometrogram of the MS Bladder

You already know the probable result of cystometry for an MS bladder. The main question is whether there will be more spasticity or more flaccidity.

The residual urine volume is usually increased. The pressure remains at zero until shortly after the residual urine volume has been reached. This first portion of the curve resembles a flaccid bladder.

Once the residual urine volume is reached during cystometry, the pressure rises rapidly. Uninhibited spasms appear. These reduce useful storage capacity and cause the sudden urgency and incontinence of spastic bladders.

Ditropan (See page 118.) inhibits bladder spasms and increases bladder storage capacity. Self-catheterization (See page 110.) and Credé (See page 106.) further increase the storage capacity by improving bladder emptying. You will benefit from these management techniques and others described in Chapter 5 if you understand the effect of spasticity and flaccidity on your own bladder function.

ANATOMY OF THE SEXUAL RESPONSE

Your entire body and your entire nervous system participate in sexual behavior. However, specific activities, like male erection and ejaculation, and female lubrication and orgasm have a more easily defined anatomical foundation.

Sexual responsiveness begins in the brain (page 258). We see, hear, or feel erotic sensations, or think erotic thoughts before any erotic response begins at genital levels. Pathways from the brain course down the brainstem and spinal cord, adjacent to the pyramidal tract (pages 313–314). They terminate in the sacral spinal cord, where special neurons control sexual activities.

Sensory Information Starts the Response

Male erection and female lubrication are *initiated* by erotic sensations or thoughts. They *occur* when spinal cord neurons are stimulated. Interruption of the pathway from brain to lower spinal cord interferes with genital responses. But interruption of this pathway for sexual expression need not interfere with erotic responses in the brain, so MSers can have and give pleasure, even though they cannot feel and move in pelvic regions.

Sensory stimulation on and near the genitals provides a powerful stimulus for sexual activity. However, normal healthy people find erogenous zones in distant parts of the body, which can initiate sexual responses as well as direct genital stimulation can. MSers and partners can use sensate focus techniques (page 261) to discover what kinds and locations of touch feel good, and which feel erotic. As the MS changes, these sites will change. MSers who remain inventive and interested can continue to find and give pleasure despite severe sensory loss.

Loss of sensitivity diminishes the immediacy of sexual pleasure. Sometimes, MSers need extra stimulation to achieve full sexual arousal. Erotic stories, erotic pictures, and erotic memories sometimes help arousal. Extra sensory stimulation of erogenous areas adds one more component.

Movement Expresses Intact Connections

Diminished movement, impotence and decreased lubrication express damaged motor pathways from the brain. These are of less importance to many people than loss of sensation. Other techniques can substitute for loss of voluntary erection and ejaculation, or loss of normal lubrication. (See Chapter 15.)

Occasionally, MSers with transverse myelitis or other local interruption of pathways to and from the brain, retain full anatomical function of their sacral spinal cord reflexes. When this happens, sensory information that normally enters via the sacral route, can provide direct reflex stimulation to sacral spinal cord autonomic neurons. This results in normal erection, normal ejaculation, and normal lubrication, but without the usual sensations perceived in the brain.

You will discover your own sexual potential if you search for it. Examine your body with your partner to discover the extent and degree of sensory loss. Discover whether you are responsive to sensory stimulation at far distant parts of your body, and whether you may perform even without sensory feedback. Concentrate on what you *can* do, more than on what you have lost. Retain joy where you find it.

Other Sensory and Motor Systems

Consider now the neurons and short fiber systems. They live in all segments of the brain and spinal cord and direct local traffic. Examine Fig. 17-2 one last time. In your mind expand that single spinal cord segment to include all the segments of the spinal cord, brainstem and brain. Think of the million sensory fibers that go to the brain, and the million motor fibers that leave it!

Each segment of the spinal cord and brainstem *receives* information from a limited area of skin, joints and muscles (which can be tested during an examination) and from other specific parts of the body (which usually cannot be tested). Each segment *sends* information to specific smooth muscles, skeletal muscles and glands.

Careful examination of muscle power and sensory function can provide detailed information about the location of plaques that affect the function of only one segment. The more you know, and especially the more your doctor knows about segmental anatomy, the better you will both understand this illness.

REFERENCES:

1) Smith, J. L.; David, N. J.: Internuclear Ophthalmoplegia. Two New Clinical Signs. *Neurology,* Minneap. Vol. 14, Pages 307–309, 1964.

Chapter 18

The Diagnosis of Multiple Sclerosis

By John K. Wolf

To establish a diagnosis of "clinically definite MS," your doctor needs three sets of information: the history, the neurological examination and the results of laboratory tests. If all three parts of the diagnostic evaluation are positive, the diagnosis of MS is more than 98% certain. Before you read further, ask yourself: how certain is your diagnosis? Did your doctor take your history with care? Was a complete neurological examination part of the diagnostic process? If your doctor is not a neurologist, have you consulted one to confirm the diagnosis? Did your physicians use established criteria to make your diagnosis? Have other possible diagnoses been considered and ruled out? Be certain that the diagnosis of MS is accurate in your case!

THE SCHUMACHER CRITERIA FOR A DIAGNOSIS OF MULTIPLE SCLEROSIS

In 1960 the National Institute for Neurological Diseases and Blindness sponsored a symposium to consider the problem of diagnosis and experimental treatment for neurological diseases. The committee on MS, chaired by Dr. George A. Schumacher, worked for the next five years. The report, called the "Schumacher committee report," hammered out six criteria for a diagnosis of "clinically definite multiple sclerosis." With small changes, these standards have been accepted by the world neurological community ever since (2).* The Schumacher criteria do not guarantee absolute accuracy of diagnosis, but if they are conscientiously applied, errors are rare.

These six criteria are complex. They discriminate between MS and other diseases that mimic MS. Let us examine each criterion in turn.

1) The Results of the Neurological Examination Must Reveal Definite Evidence of Central Nervous System Dysfunction. Symptoms Alone, No Matter How Suggestive, Cannot be Accepted as Diagnostic of Multiple Sclerosis.

Nervous people can construct a pattern of complaints that may seem similar to the history of MS, when in fact there is no organic disease at all. Neurological examinations of hysterical or nervous people are normal. Those of MSers are not. An unwary clinician, confronted with a nervous person's complaints may be tempted to say:

"Well, it *might* be multiple sclerosis!"

That comment produces anxiety, uncertainty and turmoil. It diverts patient and family from proper consideration of the nervousness and interferes with doing something about *that.*

---

*Note: References for this chapter may be found on page 345.

During a lifetime, normal people develop asymmetries of form and function which may result from handedness, accidents or diseases other than MS. Sometimes neurological examinations of normal people reveal evidence of birth defects which had not hampered their development and had previously been unrecognized. If such a person complains of neurological symptoms the examination might be abnormal, but the abnormalities would fail to explain the new complaints. On the contrary, disability caused by MS is *directly related to the location of MS plaques.*

For example, if an MSer complains of loss of vision in one eye, examination discloses decreased visual acuity, perhaps a central scotoma, abnormal pupillary responses and/or abnormal visual evoked potentials in that eye. If an MSer has "numbness from here on down," we can match the loss of one or more sensory modalities to a spinal cord lesion. The neurological examination is abnormal in direct relation to the complaint. Accurate diagnosis may follow such findings.

Do not accept a diagnosis of MS unless your physician has demonstrated unmistakable physical abnormalities that explain your symptoms. If you have doubts on this point get a second opinion.

2) There Must Be Unequivocal Evidence by History or by Examination that Two or More Discrete Parts of the Central Nervous System are Involved.

The border between MS plaque and normal tissue is distinct (Figs. 18-1, 18-2). Signs and symptoms of MS are determined by the exact location of plaques. The degree of impairment of each function depends on the degree and extent of demyelination. For the most certain

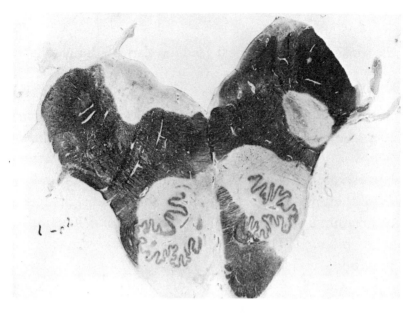

Fig.
18-1

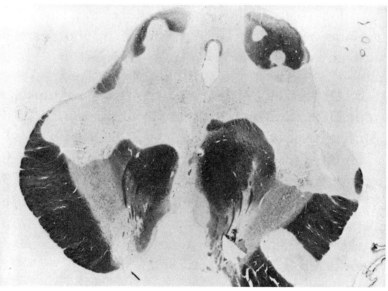

Fig.
18-2

Fig. 18-1, 18-2. Microscope slides prepared from the medulla (Fig. 18-1) and midbrain (Fig. 18-2) of a patient who died with MS. Dark areas are normally myelinated tissue. White areas are demyelinated MS plaques. Note the sharp borders between plaque and normal tissue. Distinct demarcation between plaque and normal tissue produces discrete signs on examination. Photographs courtesy of Dr. George Collins, Department of Pathology, Upstate Medical Center, Syracuse, N.Y.

diagnosis of MS it is best to demonstrate damage to at least two different levels of the central nervous system. Thus in the example above, loss of vision in one eye during an attack of optic neuritis can occur only if there is a plaque in one optic nerve. If there is numbness below a level on the trunk, there is a plaque at the corresponding level of the spinal cord, far removed from the optic nerve. Other symptoms and signs found on examination establish the presence and location of other plaques. Thus the diagnosis of *multiple* sclerosis may be established.

Ask questions as the neurologist considers your diagnosis. Be certain that your doctor has considered the question of multiple discrete lesions and has found definite evidence of their presence in your nervous system.

3) Objective evidence of Central Nervous System Disease Must Reflect Predominantly White Matter Involvement.

Multiple sclerosis attacks the myelin covering of the axons of the central nervous system. (See page 305.) These axons form the bulk of the white matter of the brain and spinal cord. Most plaques occur in the white matter. In Chapter 17 we discuss symptoms that result from damage to long tracts within the white matter of the central nervous system.

Seizures and dementia are uncommon, even in advanced MS because these are symptoms of diseased cell bodies, not diseased myelin. Neurons largely escape the effects of MS.

4) Neurological Involvement Must Occur Over a Period of Time, Either as Two Distinct Attacks Separated by At Least a Month, or by a Stepwise Progression Over a Period of At Least Six Months.

This criterion discourages a diagnosis of "clinically definite MS" during the first attack, even though the symptoms may strongly suggest it. During the first clinical attack, the CT scan, or the visual evoked potentials may demonstrate that previous attacks have already occurred without clinical symptoms. In such a case the diagnosis of MS may be considered more strongly. Even so, the six month rule is a good one to follow.

5) The First Symptom Must Have Occurred Between the Ages of 10 and 50 Years.

While it is true that MS may begin within this entire age range, or even much later in life, most MSers have their first symptom between 20 and 40.

If your first symptom occurred before age 20 or after age 40, yours is an unusual case. Be cautious about accepting the diagnosis if, for *any* reason, yours is an unusual case. Perhaps some other diagnosis could better explain your symptoms.

6) The Patient's Signs and Symptoms Cannot be Better Explained by Another Process, a Decision which Must Be Made by a Physician Competent in Clinical Neurology.

There are two reasons why a diagnosis of MS should be made by a clinical neurologist. First, neurologists are better equipped to discover evidence of some other neurological disease that might respond to specific treatment. Second, neurologists have the most experience in management of MS and other neurological diseases.

You would not accept a plumber's diagnosis on your car. Treat your body with as much respect. Consult a neurologist about neurological disease. If you are still uneasy or dissatisfied, get another opinion.

Other Clinical Criteria for the Diagnosis: "Possible MS" and "Probable MS"

The Schumacher Committee's criteria for a diagnosis of "clinically definite MS" work well for most patients and doctors. However, there are still a few patients who fit the criteria but do not have MS. Many more fail to fit the criteria but *do* have MS. This latter group has not yet had enough experience with the disease to establish the diagnosis with certainty.

On the basis of the less rigid criteria that have evolved in recent years, such people are often labeled as having "possible MS" or "probable MS." These criteria are useful in analysis of research results, but they give the individual practitioner a misleading sense of confidence that a diagnosis is at hand.

My own prejudice is not to diagnose MS if patients do not fit criteria for "clinically definite MS," and I have not yet discovered some other disease. I print in large letters on the front of the chart:

"Watch out. No diagnosis yet!"

If the person has MS, the diagnosis will become evident in time. If not, patient and doctor will be more alert to symptoms that point toward a different neurological disorder. If the undiagnosed person does have MS, there is no harm in waiting for the complete picture to develop. There is no curative treatment against MS anyway. In the meantime, the person can learn how to manage disabilities already present.

On the other hand, consider the person who has some other illness. If, during the first interview, criteria for a diagnosis of "possible MS" are met, how easy it is to accept further symptoms as confirmation of MS. Then how deep the trap when, perhaps much later, the true nature of the disease finally demands attention.

Remember, too, the nervous or fearful person, for whom the physician's statement: "Well, it *might* be MS" delays effective personal or family counseling.

With the diagnosis of "possible MS," "probable MS" or "Well, it *might* be MS," you may or may not have MS. If neither the history nor the neurological examination provide adequate evidence of MS, the physician will order laboratory examinations. When the diagnosis is doubtful, laboratory examinations can clinch the diagnosis one way or the other. That is the prime function of the laboratory: confirmation or denial.

LABORATORY EXAMINATIONS MAY CONFIRM THE DIAGNOSIS OF MS, AND CAN PROVIDE EVIDENCE FOR ILLNESSES THAT ARE NOT MS

Even though the Schumacher Committee Report was published in the dark ages of 1965 that report is still valid. MS is diagnosed at the bedside or in the office, and the diagnosis is confirmed by testing.

Modern laboratory techniques increase the reliability of diagnosis. Scientific information about the physical and chemical characteristics of MS have generated these examinations. Today we use computer technology and sensitive radiographic and biochemical techniques. Let us now consider the most important of these advances.

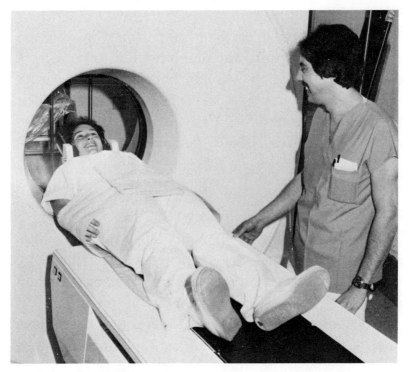

Fig. 18-3. Radiological technologists, Sue Baran, and Mike Formikell demonstrate the CT scanner. The examination is safe and informative. Patients often fall asleep as they are scanned. Photograph courtesy of the Department of Radiology, Upstate Medical Center, Syracuse, N.Y.

Computed Tomography
(CAT Scan, or CT Scan)

The CT scanner sends X-ray beams through the head in many directions on a single plane (Fig. 18-3). As these beams emerge, they are detected by sensors that transmit the information to a computer. Imagine hundreds of such beams passing through the head. The total number of these beams passing through each point are analyzed by the computer and given a numerical X-ray density. The computer does this sequentially for each point in the slice of tissue, and produces a composite picture. This is your CT scan.

The value of the CT scanner may be enhanced by contrast agents that block X-rays. When they are injected into a vein, blood vessels in the brain are visible. When injected into the spinal fluid we see the surface outline of the brain, brainstem and spinal cord. Such "contrast enhanced CT scans" disclose details of body structure that were never before visualized during life.

CT scanning safely and painlessly produces clear images of the brain. The scanner assures patient and physician that diseases have not been missed, that might alter the structure of the brain. Furthermore, the scanner may demonstrate the lesions of MS and allows patient and physician to visualize the evolution of the disease process. If the Schumacher criteria are used carefully, and the CT scanner provides diagnostic pictures (Figs. 18-4–18-6), the diagnosis will be accurate.

Magnetic Resonance Imaging

Magnetic Resonance Imaging (MRI), the latest and most sensitive diagnostic technology available to MSers, has revolutionized MS diagnosis. MRI depends on the magnetic characteristics of hydrogen atoms in water molecules. When these are exposed to a constant magnetic field, and then to a brief pulse of radio frequency energy, they give off a brief detectable electromagnetic pulse. The size of this pulse is proportional to the water concentration. Because different parts of the brain have different concentrations of water, they generate electromagnetic pulses of different magnitudes. These pulses

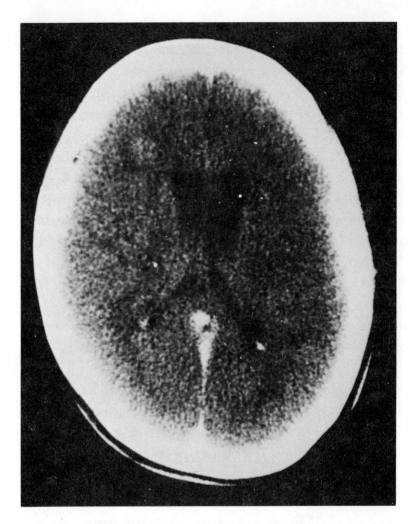

Fig. 18-4. CT scan early in the course of rapidly progressing MS. Note the enhancing lesion, top left. This is newly formed, active MS plaque.

are detected by sensors, which send the information to a computer. Computer programs determine the source of various components of the pulse. This information generates an image of the water distribution within a slice of brain, just as the CT scan computer forms an image of the X-ray densities within a slice of brain.

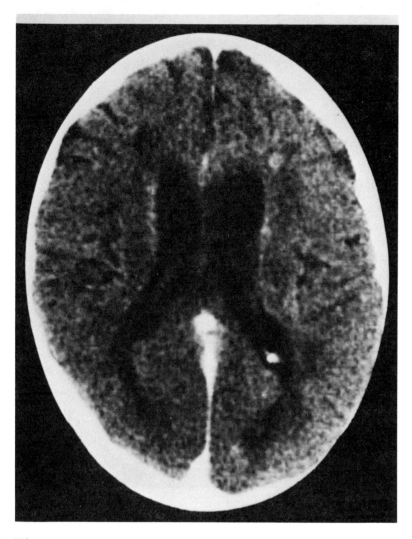

Fig. 18-5. The same woman, two months later. The acute plaque of Fig. 18-4 no longer enhances, but is visible as a darker area because of lost myelin. A new plaque has formed opposite the first, and several others near the ventricles.

As CT scanning improved, diagnosis of MS improved. For the first time in history, CT scanners displayed images of MS plaques in living subjects. Even so, CT scans of many MSers remain normal. Because of the

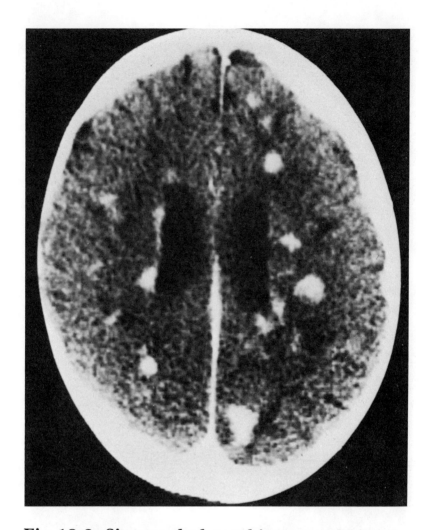

Fig. 18-6. Six months later this woman's disease has progressed rapidly. Many plaques are visible. Active plaques enhance. Older, quiescent ones are dark. CT scan photographs courtesy of the Department of Radiology, Upstate Medical Center, Syracuse, N.Y.

increased sensitivity of the new technique, MRI scans of such patients may be grossly abnormal (Fig. 18-7–18-11). MRI is much more sensitive than the best CT

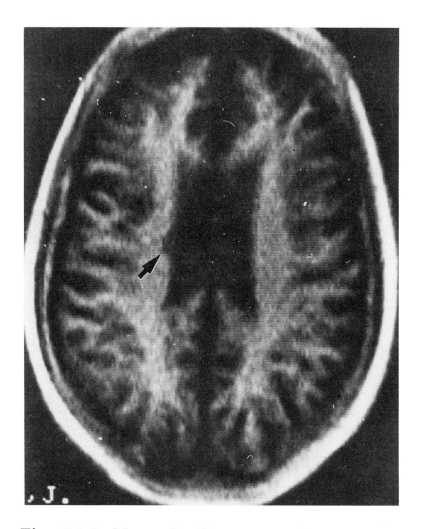

Fig. 18-7. Magnetic Resonance Image (NMR scan, or MRI) of very slowly progressive MS. All other tests were normal. Arrow points to a plaque on the ventricular surface. Another plaque is in the white matter at the other end of the arrow.

scan. Indeed, an abnormal MRI that documents the characteristic findings of MS may be added to the Schumacher criteria for a clinically definite diagnosis of MS. Some MSers have normal MRI. But they are a small minority. If the MRI is still normal, consider once more: What other diagnoses could explain the symptoms and signs?

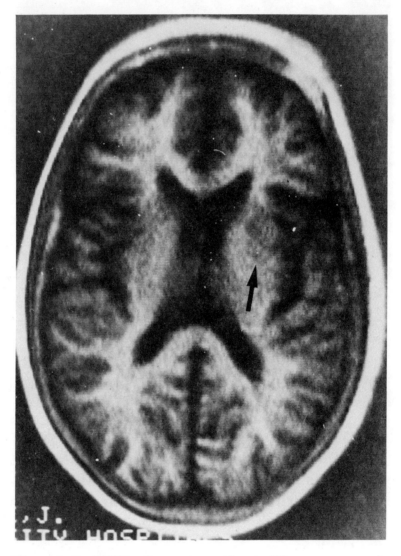

Fig. 18-8. MRI of same patient. Plaques are visible on both sides deeper in the brain. The arrow points to the most obvious one.

Fig. 18-9, 18-10; 18-11. A small change in technique makes MS plaques even more obvious on MRI. These photographs were taken from another MSer with very mild physical symptoms and complaints.

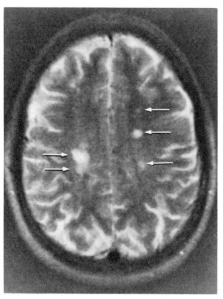

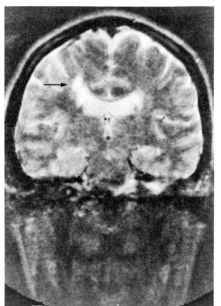

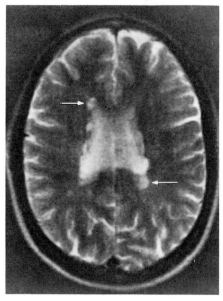

Spinal Fluid Examinations

Too much gamma globulin is produced in MS brains. In the future, when we discover the cause of this disease, we hope to understand these abnormalities of immune proteins. Now we use them as a clue to the diagnosis of MS. We look for an increased percentage of gamma globulin in the spinal fluid and for oligoclonal bands.

Oligoclonal bands? If water is removed from normal spinal fluid, and the concentrated fluid is then placed on material like filter paper and exposed to electric current, the gamma globulins spread diffusely across the display. In MSers there are often several distinct bands of gamma globulins. These represent antibody proteins that have been produced in the plaques (Fig. 18-12). During early stages of the disease some MSers have normal electrophoretic patterns and normal gamma

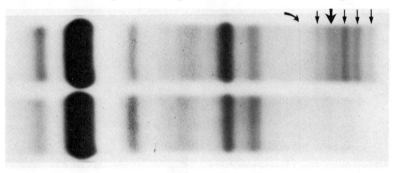

Fig. 18-12. Spinal fluid electrophoresis. Concentrated spinal fluid was applied at the curved arrow (farthest left). Albumins migrated left. Globulins migrated right. Five distinct globulin bands are visible. These are the "oligoclonal bands" of MS. Photograph courtesy of Dr. Peter Howanitz, Department of Clinical Pathology, Upstate Medical Center, Syracuse, N.Y.

globulins. Some MSers never develop detectable changes in spinal fluid. For them the diagnosis of "clinically definite MS" is made strictly by the Schumacher criteria, the CT and MRI scans and other laboratory tests.

Although increased gamma globulin and oligoclonal bands are common among MSers, they are not limited to MSers. Several other illnesses are associated with oligoclonal bands in the spinal fluid. The laboratory result can reinforce a clinical diagnosis of MS, but not establish the diagnosis by itself. For this reason, spinal tap is not a required procedure for every MS candidate. On the other hand if a myelogram is indicated to rule out other disease, or if there is another good reason for doing a spinal tap, the results of these tests may clinch the diagnosis.

Evoked Potentials

There are three kinds of evoked potentials: visual, auditory and somatosensory. For each, electrodes (buttons with wires attached) are pasted on the scalp. To record visual evoked potentials, the technician flashes a light in your eyes and the machine times the electrical response as the message reaches the visual cortex of the brain. If there is demyelination in the visual pathways, the signal will be delayed (Fig. 18-13). Sometimes this test shows this abnormality in MSers who have never had loss of vision (1). Auditory (hearing) and somatic (body sensation) evoked potentials can demonstrate demyelination in other pathways of the brainstem and spinal cord.

Discovery of abnormal evoked potentials can provide evidence of previously undetected disease in another

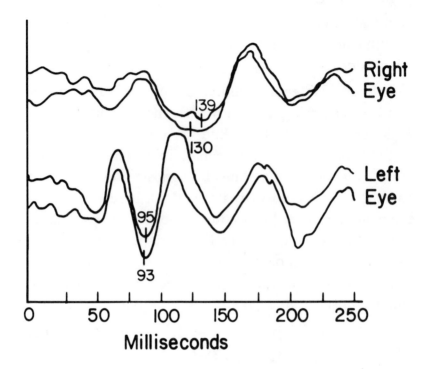

Fig. 18-13. Visual evoked potential recordings from a patient with previous optic neuritis in the right eye. The response is delayed on the right because of demyelination in that optic nerve.

region of white matter. This new clue could permit a diagnosis of "clinically definite MS" for a person whose symptoms and signs have suggested the diagnosis, but until now lacked objective proof of multiple lesions.

AFTER THE DIAGNOSIS

If there is a suspicion of a second illness, your neurologist will recommend other laboratory examinations, and, occasionally, repetition of earlier ones. A new technique like the MRI scan may confirm the diagnosis.

Use judgment in asking for such examinations. They are expensive. None of them can establish a diagnosis of MS without an adequate clinical history and physical examination. If your case is clear-cut, perhaps *no* laboratory examinations are necessary. If your diagnosis is in doubt, an examination with newly developed techniques might establish the diagnosis of MS, or establish that MS is not what was wrong in the first place.

REFERENCES:

1) Kupersmith, M. J.; Nelson, J. I.; Seiple, W. H.; Carr, R. E.; Weiss, P. A.: The 20/20 Eye in Multiple Sclerosis. *Neurology*. Vol 33, Pages 1015–1020, 1983.

2) Schumacher, G. A.; Beebe, G.; Kibler, R. F.; Kurland, L. T.; Kurtzke, J. F.; McDowell, F.; Nagler, B.; Sibley, W. A.; Tourtellotte, W. W.; Willmon, T. L.: Problems of Experimental Trials of Therapy in Multiple Sclerosis: Report by the Panel on the Evaluation of Experimental Trials of Therapy in Multiple Sclerosis. *Ann. N. Y. Acad. Sci.* Vol. 122, Pages 552–568, 1965.

Chapter 19

The Prognosis of Multiple Sclerosis
By John K. Wolf

We physicians do not usually talk about the prognosis of MS. We have been taught that it is unpredictable. This belief probably reflects the unpredictable timing of the next acute *exacerbation*. Actually, to a large degree, the general course of MS *is* predictable, even though exacerbations are not.

There is a wide spectrum of severity among MSers. About 20% have a mild course. Some remain stable for many years. Progression in most cases is slow enough so that MSers can adjust and continue to live productive lives. For the 10–15 per cent who have rapidly progressive MS, it is a terrible disease. But painful as it may be, even rapidly progressive disability is easier to bear if you plan for it.

COMPUTED PREDICTABILITY WITH TORBEN FOG

Two major studies of long term prognosis require careful examination. The first was published in 1970 by Torben Fog (2)*, who followed 73 MSers at regular

*Note: References for this chapter may be found on page 357.

intervals over a period of years. He recorded the results of examinations on a numerical scale and graphed a "disability score." On his graphs, exacerbations appear as sudden peaks in a line that showed a long-term predictable course (Figs. 19-1 and 19-2). Some of Fog's patients rapidly became disabled. Others maintained stable disability scores over many years. *None showed sudden changes in the overall course of the illness.* Fog graphed his disability scores and entered the results into a computer. It drew lines of progression similar to those illustrated in the figures. He then asked the computer two questions:

1) Based on the course as observed, what was the date of onset? The computer's analysis matched the patients' histories.

2) Based on the past history of progression, what will the disability score be in three years? In 91 percent of cases, the computer's prediction was accurate.

Some of Fog's graphs display steady progression. Others follow an exponential course, usually accelerating with the passage of time. In a few cases Fog's exponential curve showed rapid progression at the onset of the disease which stabilized with time, that is, The MS stopped progressing.

Fog's results indicate that MSers may not be able to make straight-line predictions for the next 20 years, because the course may accelerate in the future. However, Fog did show that it is possible to predict for several years ahead, because MS does not change its course suddenly. He dispelled two other false beliefs:

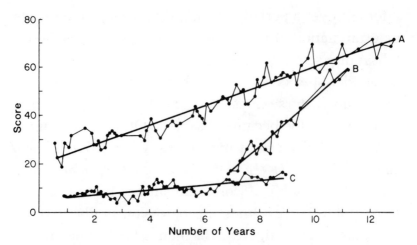

Fig. 19-1. Linear progression curves, modified from Fog (2). Case A developed slowly progressive disability during nearly 12 years of observation. Case B rapidly became disabled. Case C had hardly any progression during eight years of observation.

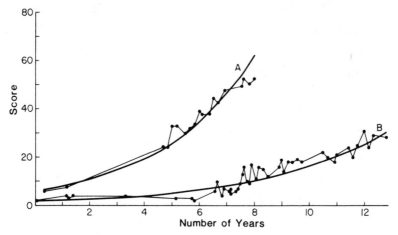

Fig. 19-2. Exponential progression curves. Both cases show an accelerating but still predictable course. Even with exponential progression, there are no sudden surprises. Note in Figs. 19-1 and 19-2, that progression does not depend on the occurrence or the severity of exacerbations.

That MS prognosis is determined by severity and frequency of exacerbations, and that prognosis is affected by age of onset.

1) MS Exacerbations Do Not Determine Prognosis.

Acute exacerbations have always been the most dramatic feature of MS. Because we think primarily in terms of exacerbations we believe they cause the progression of disability. Fog's graphs show that this is false: disability scores continued to change between attacks. After an attack, the disability score returned to the baseline of the progression curve, proving that attacks do not determine the overall severity of the *disease.*

2) Age of Onset Does Not Determine Prognosis.

Fog also confirmed the belief that late-onset MS (after 35) has fewer exacerbations and remissions. More often such patients have steadily progressive symptoms without exacerbations, but their *prognosis* was the same! Since exacerbations do not cause progression, older MSers can relax a little. Unlike their younger colleagues, they will not have sudden exacerbations, nor are they more likely to suffer rapidly progressing disability.

THE VETERAN'S ADMINISTRATION STUDY CONFIRMS AND EXPANDS FOG'S FINDINGS

Fog's study recorded frequent examinations of a few patients. The V.A. study analyzed statistics of 762 veterans, studied intensely at infrequent intervals for more than 30 years.

After careful screening to be certain they really had MS, male Army personnel were accepted into the study if they had been diagnosed while on active duty between 1942 and 1951 (7). Their lives have provided important information about the natural course of MS. Four major conclusions bear directly on prognosis.

1) Only the Previous Course of the Illness Has Predictive Value.

Like Fog, neurologists who supervised the V.A. study developed a numerical disability score. MSers in the study were questioned and examined at five year intervals after their first symptom. Many factors were analyzed in the hope of discovering which ones might be predictive of later disability.

Of all the factors examined only one was important: *the disability score at the fifth year* (3). Subjects who had minimal disability at the end of five years continued on a benign course. Those with severe disability at five years continued to have severe and progressive disease for the rest of their lives. This result is similar to Fog's. The difference is that Fog recognized the possibility of both acceleration and deceleration of progression.

These two studies indicate that if you are in the first year or so of the illness, you do not yet have enough information to make an accurate prediction. They also demonstrate that if you are a senior MSer, you may use your experience. How much disability do you have now? How much did you have several years ago? Consider the specific things you can no longer do, as well as the general course of the illness. Then look ahead a few years to estimate your own prognosis.

2) Specific Symptoms Have No Value in Predicting the Future Course of Disability.

Doctors and patients worry unnecessarily about the frequency of attacks in early years, and about peak severity of individual attacks. If bowels and bladder, or if brainstem structures are involved, we shake our heads in dismay. The Veteran's Administration study showed clearly that the degree of disability during an attack, the frequency of attacks, and specific symptoms during attacks, are of no importance in the long term prediction of disability scores.

Therefore if you are caught in the midst of an attack that seems never to end, and if you have previously experienced good remissions after other exacerbations, take courage. From that experience you can predict eventual remission this time too, knowing that only the progress of your *baseline* disability determines the prognosis.

3) There is a Definite Prognosis for Symptoms that Appear During an Attack.

It is cold comfort to the MSer, caught in a seemingly endless attack, to know that disability progresses independently of attacks. At that moment there are more important questions: How long will this attack last? How permanent are these symptoms? Can someone predict the eventual outcome of this attack?

There is no specific answer for an individual attack, but statistical information may be useful. J. F. Kurtzke, who played a prominent role in the formal V.A. study, asked of veterans in his hospital: What is the prognosis of individual symptoms that have been present for two years or less?

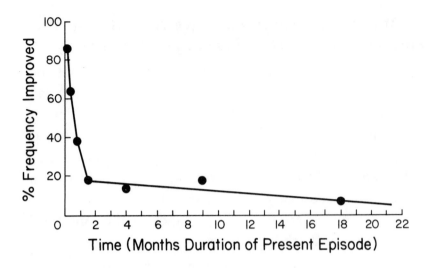

Fig. 19-3. The course of individual symptoms may be predicted from their duration at the time of observation. New symptoms are likely to remit. Old symptoms are probably permanent. Modified from Kurtzke (3).

After considering many factors, he found that only the *duration* of a symptom determined the statistical chance of its disappearance (4). If a symptom has been present for only a week, there is an 86% chance that it will go away. If it has been present for a month, there is a 38% chance of disappearance. Symptoms present for two years or more are probably permanent (Fig. 19-3).

These statistics parallel the daily experience of MSers. They have "bad days" when a leg refuses to walk properly or fatigue turns to exhaustion. On such a day the MSer can look to tomorrow with fair assurance that it will be better. MSers usually do not call the doctor to report an exacerbation until a new symptom has persisted for a week or more, and is accompanied by other symptoms that indicate this is not merely a "bad week."

This hesitation may reflect an unwillingness to admit to another exacerbation. However, it is more likely the result of past experience with symptoms that went away on their own.

4) Optic Neuritis is Not a Sure Sign of Multiple Sclerosis.

Many patients with optic neuritis have been told that they have a 30–50% chance of getting MS. The V.A. study demonstrated that the risk is less.

Male Army personnel who developed only optic neuritis while on active duty were included in this part of the study (6). Excluded were those who developed optic neuritis and other neurological symptoms, and those who developed a second bout of optic neuritis within a few weeks of the first. Optic neuritis, associated with other neurological symptoms, and repeated optic neuritis, are common early symptoms of MS.

After 12 to 18 years of observation, only 12 percent of the study group had developed clinically definite MS. By projecting their data into the future the authors expected that a maximum of 19 percent of patients with isolated optic neuritis would ever develop MS.

The significance and even the basic nature of optic neuritis continue to be controversial. Two brief articles outline the issues. Each has an extensive bibliography to lead you further into the literature (1, 5).

The V.A. study was an enormous and comprehensive examination of the natural history of MS. I have presented only those parts of the study that deal with prognosis. If you wish to read the rest of the V.A. study your librarian can help you find other articles in the series.

WEATHER AND BODY TEMPERATURE HAVE PREDICTABLE EFFECTS ON MS SYMPTOMS

Weather and climate have little effect on the long term course of MS. However, the weather affects the well-being of many MSers. Spring and summer are hard times. When the weather begins to change in May, neurologists' phones begin to ring. MSers have deteriorated. They are tired and walk poorly. They have more flexor spasms. They wonder if this is another attack. A second epidemic of exhaustion occurs in July and August when the summer heat beats down.

Increase in body temperature is such an adverse factor for MSers that in former years the hot water bath became a diagnostic test. On the other hand, too cool a body temperature may also aggravate muscle spasms and interfere with walking because of increased spasticity. Such functional changes last longer than the one afternoon of being overheated or chilled, but they do not represent an acute exacerbation of MS.

During hot weather, or during an illness accompanied by fever, MSers should try to stay cool. Use air conditioners, frequent dips in a swimming pool or a cool bath. If necessary, take aspirin or Tylenol® to reduce fever, and antibiotics to eradicate bacterial infections.

If overcooling in winter worsens spasms, dress more warmly, exercise more and use more of the antispastic medications described in Chapter 4.

PREGNANCY PROBABLY HAS NO EFFECT ON PROGNOSIS

Men and women have about the same chance of developing slowly or rapidly progressive disability. A recent article by Poser and Poser reviews the previous literature and presents their analysis of the course of MS among 512 women who responded to a questionnaire (8). They found that pregnancy does not affect prognosis.

My own experience with MSers and their families suggests that MS adds just one more factor to the many stresses that affect all families. We all worry about money, jobs, sex, about our kids and about other people in our lives. Sometimes MS is a major problem, but strong families survive. Weak ones fail. Some MSer marriages that would have succeeded without the added burden of MS *or* growing children fail because of the combination. I do not know how a couple can tell in advance that their marriage will succeed.

When deciding for or against a pregnancy, consider this: Children of strong MS families emerge fortified by the experiences of success despite adversity. Those children may have a stormier adolescence than if they had grown up in families without chronic illness. Such storms break hearts at the time, but the storms of adolescence are not the same as failed lives. Read Verah Johnson's Prologue.

Examine the long-term issues of a pregnancy. Look at the course of your MS to this point. If you have three to five years of experience you can make an approximate prediction of your future course. Read once more Mitzi's chapters on parents, children and spouses (pages 214–253). Talk with senior MSers about their experiences.

Above all, think together as a couple about the strengths and weaknesses of your marriage. Think together about how strongly each of you wants children. If you think you can learn important things about yourselves and your marriage from a family counselor, find someone to help you learn together.

Assemble all the information you can. Make the best possible decision about a pregnancy, and act on it. Whatever your conclusion, there will be times when you regret that decision. But informed decisions are far better than those made during emotional turmoil, or non-decisions that happen by default.

SUMMARY

For some readers this chapter will have proven painful, because it confirmed inner knowledge they already had: that theirs is a rapidly progressive case of MS. For others, the chapter will be less painful.

There is no choice about the future course of this illness. But we have many choices about how we manage its symptoms and our lives. MSers can plan ahead to cope with individual disabling symptoms as they arise. If your disease has progressed rapidly, you can plan how you will respond to advancing disability. If your job is threatened during an attack of MS and you know that the progress of your disease is slow or moderate, you have statistics to help you fight harder to keep your job. You can plan in your younger years to be a capable spouse and parent despite changing symptoms and changing family needs.

Healthy or sick, we all have the same problem: management. Healthy people must learn to manage the progressive disabilities of aging. MSers must learn to manage the combination of aging plus MS. I have no illusions that even the best of regimens and the brightest of ideas can offer perfection. However, if ideas about management allow you to remain an active productive citizen despite this disease, you have been successful!

REFERENCES:

1) Ebers, G. C.: Optic Neuritis and Multiple Sclerosis. *Arch. Neurol.* Vol. 42, Pages 702–704, 1985.

2) Fog, T.: The course of Multiple Sclerosis in 73 Cases with Computer-Designed Curves. *Acta Neurol. Scand.* Vol. 46 (Suppl. 47), 1970.

3) Kurtzke, J. F.; Beebe, G. W.; Nagler, B.; Kurland, L. T.; Auth, T. L.: Studies on the Natural History of Multiple Sclerosis; 8. Early Prognostic Features of the later course of the illness. *J. Chron. Dis.* Vol 30, Pages 817–830, 1977.

4) Kurtzke, J. F.: Course of Exacerbations of Multiple Sclerosis in Hospitalized Patients. *Arch. Neurol., Psychiat.* Vol 76, Pages 175–184, 1956.

5) Kurtzke, J. F.: Optic Neuritis and Multiple Sclerosis. *Arch. Neurol.* Vol. 42, pages 704–710, 1985.

6) Kurland, L. T.; Beebe, G. W.; Kurtzke, J. F.; Nagler, B.; Auth, T. L.; Lessell, S.; Nefzger, M. D.: Studies on the Natural History of Multiple Sclerosis; 2. The Progression of Optic Neuritis to Multiple Sclerosis. *Acta Neurol. Scand.* Vol 41 (Suppl. 16), pages 157–176, 1965.

7) Nagler, B.; Beebe, G. W.; Kurtzke, J. F.; Kurland, L. T.; Auth, T. L.; Nefzger, M. D.: Studies on the Natural History of Multiple Sclerosis; 1. Design and Diagnosis. *Acta Neurol. Scand.* Vol 42 (Suppl 19), Pages 141–156, 1966.

8) Poser, S.; Poser, W.: Multiple Sclerosis and Gestation. *Neurology* Vol. 33, Pages 1422–1427, 1983.

Chapter 20
Research *vs.* Quackery
The Exploitation of Hope
By John K. Wolf

Since 1963 I have watched MSers travel from one "promising treatment" to the next, always hoping that this will be the one. I have even prescribed some of those treatments with the same hope. As a neurology resident I prescribed histamine drips, and later for a year, Orinase®. Now we use ACTH and Prednisone, and in desperate straights we try immunosuppressants. At this writing, no useful treatment for long-term improvement of multiple sclerosis exists. We continue to wait.

Meanwhile, I *look* for the opportunity to prescribe medications like Lioresal®, Elavil® and Ditropan®, because these medications help MSers live better. I look for aids to mobility and I am pleased when they make life easier. But MSers regard these remedies as peripheral. They want a cure. The issue we face today is not cure, but management. Management is the central theme of this book.

QUACKERY

While researchers grope slowly toward the cause and possible cure of MS, quacks flourish and become wealthy. The essence of quackery is dishonesty. The number of college degrees, and current affiliation with institutions of any kind are irrelevant, if the motive is mercenary. Quacks offer new and "promising" treatments for chronic disabling diseases, but their purpose is money, not the eradication of suffering.

There is no sure-fire formula for distinguishing quacks and their quackery from legitimate practitioners. However, I have formulated 10 characteristics of quackery that may help you. Use them as you assess the person and the program, and make your own diagnosis.

Criteria of Quackery

1) Quack treatments are announced in the press, on television "news" programs and by word of mouth, not by reports to legitimate medical meetings, nor in reputable medical journals.

2) Quacks often imply that their new treatment is based on recent "research." It is often based on some shred of legitimate medical evidence, but the treatment is "promising" before the shred has proved important.

3) Quack treatments are available to anyone who can pay. There is no effort to control results, to collect accurate data, to document success or failure.

Look at the result of placebo treatment for MS exacerbations. Note that 69% were improved after four weeks (page 190). Look at Kurtzke's work to see the natural course of MS symptoms (page 351). Look at your own history and remember how often you have improved after you had gotten worse. Then ask if your prospective treatment has been evaluated against this background of the known course of MS.

4) When questioned, the quack produces testimonials from someone previously duped, who praises the work and indicates great improvement after treatment. Beware the bearer of testimonials. He is not a scientist. He is almost always a quack.

5) Quackery is expensive. Few legitimate treatments for MS cost several thousand dollars for a couple of weeks of outpatient evaluation and some shots or pills. Successful quacks justify the fee by claiming to support a vast research effort that does not exist.

6) Quacks use self-aggrandizement to attract gullible people. Their press releases and letters to patients are phrased in medical jargon that out-Greeks and out-Latins the fanciest medical writers. One brochure indicated that the doctor had been nominated for the Nobel Prize: "nominated," not "awarded." I hereby nominate the reader of this paragraph for the Nobel Prize in the Reading of Great Literature and assign the spouse—or anyone else—to write the letter of recommendation to Stockholm.

7) Quacks guard their treatments jealously. They claim either that they are so new that they must first be evaluated, or that an interfering government prevents general use. This second ploy appeals to our universal and healthy distrust of government. The result in either case is that neither the "research"—nor the income— can be disseminated.

8) The double-talk and double-write of quackery fosters false hopes. Quack claims are indistinct and irresistible. They make no promise of cure, only "relief," but the words are phrased imprecisely so the hope of cure is never abandoned.

If the literature you read raises you to a fever pitch, If you feel you must write or phone immediately—hang the expense!—sit back for a moment and analyze the message. Reread the brochure for facts, evidence and data. Compare the brochure with this ten-point list.

9) Successful quacks are really nice guys. They impress patients with their kindness and concern.

> "He was one of the sweetest people I have ever met."
> "—Totally dedicated to his work"
> "—Showed more concern for me and my welfare than anyone I have ever met!"

> "But his business manager is really nasty. He demanded payment in advance, refused us credit and badgered us about future payments."

When did you last meet this team? Think of your recent automobile purchase. The salesman was pleasant and interested while you made your deal, the irritable manager ruthless as he raised your price. Those two worked well together. Their dance was carefully planned and beautifully executed. If you left with a car and a good deal, you were proud of yourself.

Think of the kindly resort owner who took you to the secret fishing spots and showed you a fantastic time. It was the unpleasant partner who tacked on the extra charges for every moment spent. These combinations do not occur by accident! The "second" never does a thing the "first" really dislikes.

Although quack and business manager "fight" throughout the week, Friday evening after work they meet for dinner, or sip martinis on the afterdeck, surrounded by blue water and cooled by gentle breezes. They know they have found the good life. It is paid for by the money and hopes of people who have come to them for help. The scam has worked, and the martinis are excellent!

10) Last, the quack makes no effort to establish an accurate diagnosis before beginning treatment. Everyone gets about the same treatment, assured that it is "tailored to individual needs." This is an especially sticky problem for MSers. The diagnosis of MS cannot be established with perfect confidence anyway, and they know it. But any new therapy must be *established* by treatment of patients with the best documentation possible!

Some of my MSers went to Washington, D.C. for acupuncture in the mid-1970's. It was the raging fad then. They came home impressed with the extensive medical history and physical examination performed before they were treated. When I asked, if there had been a neurological history or examination they were startled. They had been asked "what is your diagnosis?" and were then acu-punctured for MS. This is *plain unadulterated quackery.*

MSers who have been scammed know it deep down. If you have been one of these, you may find yourself defending your scammer with unaccustomed shrillness. You may assure anyone who will listen that the treatment worked. As you return home, you may expend extra effort to come off the airplane walking.

If your friends recognize the reason for your shrillness they can avoid the scammer. If they do not, they may become grist for his mill.

If a practitioner fits these criteria, or a friend sounds too shrill, recognize the scam for what it is. If you choose to go anyway, go with realistic doubts. Spend money if you like. Money is cheap. Do not spend your hopes. They are irreplaceable.

LEGITIMATE RESEARCH

Conducting research and providing medical care are distinctly different occupations. If you live near a research center and you wish to be part of that effort, do it in the hope that your contribution will advance knowledge. Do not join a research project in the hope of better medical care, or cure. The object of research is to collect accurate data about a specific question. While you help the project, continue to live the best life possible through excellent management of your MS.

If your research project happens to test the first effective treatment for MS, you may receive direct benefit from the work. If it does not, and your participation provides one small step toward understanding of the disease, you have made an honorable contribution. Enter a research project with that limited goal in mind. Leave it later, satisfied that your participation has been important.

Recognizing the Cure

The cure for MS is not yet at hand. When it finally arrives you may recognize it by characteristics that mark legitimate advances in scientific medicine.

1) The real cure for MS will come from a group of recognized researchers. They may be biochemists or immunologists instead of neurologists. Whoever discovers it will have devoted years of hard work to the problem.

2) Funding is more likely to be governmental than private. Certainly the research will not be supported by

fee-for-service provided by thousands of individual patients.

3) Before the study begins, criteria will be established. Patients will be examined and the limited number who fit the criteria will be accepted for the research project.

4) Although MSers may first hear of the cure in the lay press, its first revelation will occur among researcher friends in the hospital cafeteria. Only after the results of the research have become more certain will reports be given at medical meetings, or published in reputable medical journals. After that, the media can inform the public.

5) The effective treatment will be universally available very soon thereafter. There will be great excitement in the neurological community. Your neurologist will be *itching* to use it or to send you somewhere to receive the treatment.

Like you, I hope the real thing will soon arrive, but I know that MSers have lived successful lives in its absence. MSers who have learned management have taught each other and their doctors how to master disability, even though they did not know how to stop their disease. Until the cure does come, continue to hope and continue to cope.

I wish you good fortune!

Glossary

Many words in this glossary are discussed in the text and redefined here. Some words that relate to MS may not appear in the text but we include them for MSers who encounter them in discussion and reading.

This glossary can become much more useful if readers write us about words that should be included. Please help to enlarge this glossary.

Acuity, Visual

Clarity of vision. Visual acuity is expressed as a fraction of normal vision. A visual acuity of 20/20 indicates an eye that sees at 20 feet what an average eye sees at 20 feet. Visual acuity of 20/400 indicates an eye that sees at 20 feet what an average eye sees at 400 feet.

Analgesic

Pain medication.

Anterior (Also Ventral)

Toward the front (standing up). Toward the belly surface of the body or of an organ.

Anterior Horn (Of the Spinal Cord)

When early anatomists examined the central gray matter of the spinal cord they thought it resembled the horns of a deer. In fig. 17-2, page 307, the anterior horn is at the bottom of the central gray matter. It contains motor neurons. The posterior horn is at the top. It contains sensory neurons.

Anterior Horn Cell (Anterior Horn Neuron)

A motor neuron in the anterior horn gray matter of the spinal cord. Anterior horn cells extend their axons directly to the muscles of the body.

Association Cortex

See Cortex, Association.

Asymmetry (Asymmetrical)

Not the same on the two sides.

Atrophy, Optic

The atrophic optic nerve appears pale when viewed through the ophthalmoscope. This is caused by loss of myelin, optic nerve fibers and blood vessels in the optic nerve.

Attack

See Exacerbation.

Axon

See Fig. 17-1 page 304. The axon conducts impulses away from the dendritic zone.

Babinski's Sign (After Joseph Babinski, French Neurologist, 1857–1932)

Babinski lived and worked in Paris during an exciting time of discovery in clinical neurology. He described many clinical signs, but Babinski's Toe Sign is the most important. When the sole of the foot is scratched, the big toe goes up and the little toes spread apart. Presence of Babinski's sign means there is damage to the corticospinal tract somewhere between the brain and the lower spinal cord. See page 314.

Biochemistry

Study of the chemistry of living organisms.

Biological Half-Life

See Half-Life, Biological.

Bout

See Exacerbation.

Brainstem

See Fig. 17-3, page 310. The brainstem connects the brain to the spinal cord. It has three major parts, the midbrain, pons and medulla.

Bundle (In the Central Nervous System)

See Tract.

Cell Membrane

The thin layer of proteins, fats and carbohydrates, which forms the "outside skin" of the cell.

Central Nervous System

See Nervous System, Central.

Cerebellum

See Fig. 17-3, page 310 and discussion, page 315. The cerebellum lies on top of the brainstem. Its chief functions concern balance and coordination of movement.

Cervical

See segment.

Clinician

A health professional especially trained in diagnosis and management of disease.

Clonus

Rapidly alternating involuntary contraction and relaxation of a muscle. Ankle clonus is the most common form of clonus. Contraction and relaxation of calf muscles at the ankle makes the foot and leg bounce up and down. Clonus is a symptom of spasticity.

Column (Of the Spinal Cord)

See Tract.

Cortex (From Latin, Meaning Bark or Rind)

The outer layer of an organ.

Cortex, Association

The cortex immediately adjacent to and closely connected to the primary sensory cortex. Association cortex gives form and meaning to sensory messages.

368

Cortex, Cerebral

The outer layers of nerve cells that cover the entire surface of the cerebral hemispheres. Thinking and other complex neuronal activities occur in the cerebral cortex.

Corticospinal Tract

See Tract, Corticospinal.

Credé (After Karl Credé, a German Gynecologist, 1847–1929)

Credé devised a procedure to force the placenta from the uterus immediately after birth. By squeezing the uterus, he forced it down into the pelvis. This same maneuver helps to empty an enlarged bladder.

CT (CAT) Scan

Computed Axial Tomography. See discussion, page 334.

Dementia

Mental deterioration.

Demyelination

Loss of the myelin sheath that normally covers nerve axons.

Dendritic Zone (Dendritic Tree)

The part of a neuron that receives nerve impulses. See discussion, pages 302–303 and fig. 17-1, page 304.

Diagnosis

The determination of the specific nature of a disease, sign or symptom. The accuracy of a particular diagnosis depends on the quality of thought and physical examination, as well as the specificity of laboratory tests.

Diffuse

See Focal

Diuretic

Water pill. A diuretic encourages the kidneys to excrete more free water and salt. Usually used to combat edema or to treat high blood pressure.

Edema

Swelling of tissues caused by water retention. Edema usually collects in feet and ankles when there is paralysis, because fluid is not pumped out of the legs by movement of the muscles.

Electrode

An attachment with a surface designed to transmit electric current. In medical practice, electrodes are usually used to connect electronic instruments to a patient's body.

Electrophoresis

A laboratory technique. Separates materials on the basis of their individual electrical charge and size.

Spinal fluid electrophoresis is used to separate proteins in the spinal fluid. Concentrated spinal fluid is applied to a starch gel or other base, and electrical current is applied across the gel. Different proteins move at different velocities in the electrical field. See Fig. 18-12, page 342.

Evoked Potentials, Visual

See discussion, page 343.

Exacerbation (Also Attack, Bout)

An abrupt increase in the severity of symptoms. An MS exacerbation usually lasts for weeks or months. During an exacerbation, numerous individual symptoms may come and go in succession.

Exacerbations are usually followed by complete or partial *Remission*; the abatement, or diminution of symptoms after an exacerbation.

Excretion

Elimination or discharge by normal means. Urine and feces are excreted.

To be distinguished from *Secretion,* which is the process of making a specific substance and releasing it for use. Saliva is secreted in the mouth. Digestive juices are secreted in the stomach.

Fasciculus

See Tract

Fasciculus, Medial Longitudinal

See discussion, page 315. The MLF is a nerve fiber tract that controls horizontal eye movements.

Flaccid

Limp, soft, weak.

To be distinguished from *spastic.* Spastic muscles may also have loss of power, but spastic muscles are more tense, harder and more reactive than normal.

Focal

Highly localized to one place.

To be distinguished from *Multifocal,* indicating several highly localized processes in different places.

Also to be distinguished from *Diffuse,* indicating a widely distributed process without definite boundaries.

Figs. 18-1 and 18-2, page 329 show evidence of multifocal MS plaques with sharp boundaries.

Gamma Globulin (Also Written as   -Globulin

Blood proteins that carry antibody activity.

White blood cells in MS plaques make gamma globulins that may be found in the spinal fluid. Increased amounts of gamma globulins and the presence of oligoclonal gamma globulin bands in the spinal fluid electrophoresis are characteristic of MS. See discussion, page 342.

Gene

The biological unit of heredity. Genes determine the structure and function of all proteins in the body. In their turn, proteins govern body shape and function.

Gland

A collection of cells that secrete materials unrelated to their own needs. For instance, the salivary gland secretes saliva. Those cells have no use for saliva, but the mouth and stomach need it for digestion.

Gray Matter

Portions of the central nervous system where nerve cell bodies are concentrated. Cortex is gray matter. So are the anterior and posterior horns of the spinal cord.

Half-Life, Biological

The time required to eliminate half the medication already present in the body. See discussion, page 87.

Hysterical Symptoms

Symptoms brought to a physician that are not caused by organic disease. The definition given here applies to the use of the word in this volume. Various authors use the same word with different meanings.

Incontinence, Overflow

Urinary incontinence due to the pressure of retained urine in an enlarged (and usually flaccid) bladder.

Lateral

Toward one side (of an organ or of the body).

Lateral Spinothalamic Tract

See Tract, Lateral Spinothalamic.

Lesion

Any abnormal damage to tissue structure or function. A scar is a lesion. So is a cancer, an MS plaque, a stomach ulcer, or a pimple.

Lobe (Of the Brain)

A major division of the cerebral hemispheres. The cerebral hemispheres are divided into frontal, parietal, temporal and occipital lobes. See Fig. 17-3, page 310.

Lumbar

See segment.

Ophthalmoscope

An instrument designed for examination of the inner structure of the eye. The ophthalmoscope has a light source to illuminate the inside of the eye, and a lens system that allows sharp focus on many portions of the eye.

Medial

Toward the middle (of an organ or of the body).

Modality

A particular kind of function, usually sensory. Sensory modalities include perception of temperature, pain, position, movement.

MRI

See discussion, page 335.

Multifocal

See focal.

Muscle, Skeletal

Striped muscles (under the microscope) that are at-tached to bones and generally cross at least one joint space. Voluntary muscles responsible for body move-ments.

Muscle, Smooth

Unstriped, involuntary muscle. Smooth muscle is found in intestines, bladder, blood vessels and other places in the body. Smooth muscle is innervated by the autonomic nervous system. See pages 316–324. In con-trast to the voluntary activity of skeletal muscles, the action of smooth muscle is always involuntary.

Myelin

Fatty substance which forms a sheath around some nerve fibers in the central and peripheral nervous systems. Myelin is formed by specialized cells and consists largely of their cell membranes which are wrapped around the axon.

Myelitis, Transverse

Symptoms that result from development of MS plaques at one spinal cord level. Transverse myelitis can cause severe loss of movement and sensation. Recovery from transverse myelitis is similar to recovery from other MS symptoms. The plaques are identical.

Nerve Impulse

The electrochemical charge carried by an axon.

Nervous System, Central

The cerebral hemispheres, brainstem, cerebellum and spinal cord.

Nervous System, Peripheral

All the nerves and nerve cells outside the central nervous system.

Neuritis, Optic (Also Papillitis and Retrobulbar Neuritis)

Inflammation of the optic nerve.
If inflammation affects the optic nerve head *in* the eye it is called *Papillitis.*
If inflammation affects the optic nerve *behind* the eye it is called *Retrobulbar Neuritis.*

Neurologist

American Neurologists have graduated from college, then medical school. They have successfully completed one year of internship and at least three years of residency training in neurology. During the first 18 months the resident cares for hospitalized neurological patients. During the second 18 months, most neurology residents learn about EEG, EMG, evoked responses, neuropathology, child neurology and other special areas. Many neurologists take the "Board Examinations" for national certification in neurology. Neurologists in other countries have similar credentials.

Neuron

Any of the conducting cells of the nervous system. See Fig. 17-1, page 304.

Neurophysiologist

Neurophysiologists usually have earned a PhD degree in neurophysiology, the study of the function of the nervous system.

NMR

Nuclear Magnetic Resonance. See discussion, page 335.

Oligoclonal Bands

See Gamma Globulin. See also discussion, page 342.

Optic Atrophy

See Atrophy, Optic.

Optic Nerve

The nerve of vision

Orbit

The bony socket for the eye.

Organelle (Means Little Organ)

Particles within cells that are covered with their own membrane. Within cells there are many different kinds of organelle, each with its own special function.

Papillitis

See Neuritis, Optic.

Paralysis

Total inability to move a part of the body because of nerve or muscle dysfunction.

Peripheral Nervous System

See Nervous System, Peripheral.

Pathway

See Tract.

Plaque

The demyelinating lesion of MS. See discussion, pages 305–306 and 328–330.

Placebo

Treatment with no therapeutic value.

Posterior (Also Dorsal)

Toward the back side of the body or of an organ.

Posterior Column

Bundle of axons in the posterior part of the spinal cord. Interruption of the posterior column on one side of the spinal cord causes loss of position sense on the same side of the body below the level of the interruption. See Fig. 17-2, page 307, discussion, page 308.

Posterior Horn

See Anterior Horn.

Prognosis

A forecast of the probable outcome of a symptom or illness.

Protein

Any of a large group of complex organic molecules composed chiefly of amino acids. Proteins govern the structure and function of all body parts.

Pyramidal Tract

See Tract, Pyramidal.

Remission

See Exacerbation

Residual Urine Volume

See Volume, Residual Urine.

Retrobulbar Neuritis

See Neuritis, Optic.

Sacral

See Segment

Scotoma (From Greek, Meaning a Dark Place)

An area of depressed or absent vision within the visual field. A *Central Scotoma* consists of loss or absence of vision in the center of the visual field. A central scotoma causes loss of visual acuity. See discussion, page 311–312.

Secretion

See Excretion.

Segment (Of Spinal Cord)

One defined portion of the spinal cord.

In the spinal cord, there are eight *Cervical* segments (neck and upper extremities), twelve *Thoracic* segments (chest and trunk), five *Lumbar* segments (lower extremities) and five *Sacral* segments (buttocks, bowel, bladder and sexual functions).

Sign (of Disease)

See Symptom.

Spastic

See Flaccid.

Symptom (Of Disease)

Any evidence of malfunction perceived by a *patient.*

A *Sign* is any evidence of malfunction perceived by an *examiner.*

Thoracic

See Segment.

Tract (In the Central Nervous System. Also Bundle, Column, Fasciculus, Pathway)

Axons traveling together. In most cases, the origin and destination of axons in a tract are quite similar.

Tract, Pyramidal (Also Corticospinal)

One of the major motor tracts of the central nervous system. The Pyramidal Tract is so-named because it passes through the pyramids of the medulla on its way from the brain to the spinal cord. See discussion, page 313.

Tract, Lateral Spinothalamic

A tract in the anterior-lateral portion of the spinal cord. Interruption of the Lateral Spinothalamic Tract results in loss of pain and temperature sensation on the opposite side of the body below the level of the interruption. See Fig. 17-2, discussion, page 306.

Ureter

The tube that conducts urine from the kidney to the bladder.

Urethra

The tube that conducts urine from the bladder to the outside of the body.

Visual Acuity

See acuity, Visual.

Visual Evoked Potential

See discussion, page 343.

Visual Field

The part of space that the fixed eye can see.

Volume, Residual Urine

The amount of urine remaining in the bladder immediately after voiding. See discussion, page 99.

White Matter

That part of the Central Nervous System containing
mostly axons, their myelin coating and supporting cells.

Index

CT (CAT) scan, use in diagnosis of MS   334–335
Culture, urine   103
Cystometrogram   319–322

D

Dantrium (dantrolene)   94–96
Depression   142–157
    antidepressant medications, Table   150–151
    vs. emotional incontinence   154–155
    insomnia caused by   207
    vs. mobility   30
    sexual dysfunction caused by   268–269
    symptoms   142–144
    treatment   144–154
Diagnosis of MS   326–345
Diagnosis, definition   370
Diazepam. See Valium
Dibenzyline   121
Dilantin, use against MS pains   167, 171
Disimpaction, manual   140–141
Ditropan   118–120
Diuretic, definition   370
Double vision, anatomy   315
Double voidings   107–108

E

Elavil use against depression   144–154
   use against MS pains   171
   use against emotional incontinence   156
Electrophoresis, definition   370–371
Elevators, for home access   48–51
Emergency supply, of medications   93
Emotional incontinence   154–156

Foot drop   20
Four-point cane   15–16

G

Gait disturbance after sexual intercourse   264
Gamma globulin, definition   372
Grandfather's cane   13–15

H

Half-life, biological   87
Hysterical, definition   373

I

I.M. injection technique   193–195
Impotence   265–266
    stuffing   265
Indwelling catheter   123–127
    sexual intercourse with   126–127
Infection, bladder   99–104
Information about MS, best sources   294
INH. See isoniazid
Injection technique, intramuscular   193–195
Insomnia, management   203–209
International travel ideas   33
Isoniazid for tremor   178–182
    best dose   181–182
    hepatitis   178–180
    indications   178
    pyridoxine prevents neuropathy   181
    side effects   178–181
    sleepiness   180–181

treatment strategy 181–182
warnings 178–181

J

Johnson, Verah, Prologue xxvii–xxx

K

Krauss, Fred, Jr., Dedication v–vi

L

Laughing and crying, inappropriate 154–156
l-DOPA, treatment for emotional
  incontinence 155–156
Lesion, definition 374
Lhermitte's sign 161–162
Lioresal 85–94
  use against tic douloureux 164–165

M

Management, goals 2
Marriage and MS 237–245
  advancing disability, effect 239–240
  anger and depression 237–239
  effect of chronic illness 238–240
  fighting for survival 240–242
  separation and divorce 243–244
  sexual relationships 242–243
Masturbation
  further reading (for women) (Barbach) 276
  further reading (for men) (Zilbergeld) 277
Mobility International U.S.A. 33
Motor functions in brain and spinal cord 313–325

gait disturbance after intercourse   264

impotence   265-266

remission, definition   371

spasticity impairs sexual function   268

worse in hot weather   354

MSer, term   8-9

Muscle, skeletal, definition   375

Muscle, smooth, definition   375

Myelin, definition   375

N

Nervousness, management   209-211

Neuritis, optic, retrobulbar, definition   376

Neurologist, definition   376

Neuron   302-306

axon   305

cell body   303-305

dendritic zone   302-303

NMR scan, use in diagnosis of MS   335-341

O

Optic atrophy, definition   366

Optic neuritis   159-160, 186

definition   376

not a sure sign of MS   353

Oxybutynin chloride   118-120

P

Pain and temperature, anatomy   306-308

Pain in MS   158-173

Lhermitte's sign   161-162

of spasticity   160-161

of weakness   160

Q

R

S

T

Tegretol   163–172
    biological half-life   171–172
    complications   168–171
    dose   171–172
    side effects   168–171
Tic douloureux   163–165
Tonic seizures   166–168
Tract, lateral spinothalamic, definition   381
    of CNS, definition   381
      medial longitudinal fasciculus   315
      posterior columns   308–311, 378
      pyramidal, definition   313, 381
Transportation, accessible   72–79
    community access   78–79
    handicapped parking   78
    private car   73–78
    public transportation   72–73
Travel, international   33
Trigeminal neuralgia   163–165

U

Urinalysis   102–103
Urinary tract infection   99–104
Urine culture   103
Urine sample, mid-stream   102
Urodynamic evaluation   117–118, 319–322

V

Valium, in treatment of spasticity   96–97
Vitamin C in bladder management   105–106
Volume, residual urine   99–100, 109

Autobiography

I never wanted to be crippled: A nurse? An actress!
Maybe a teacher.

I prepared for a life I would never live.
How could I know
My body carried multiple sclerosis?
The audacity! I just learned to dance!

So? Learn something else!

I fought. I kicked. I screamed.
(I still do sometimes.)
Finally I studied what was left of life.

I kept good childhood values like honesty.
I threw out impossible expectations.

I packed away cherished memories,
To taste from time to time.
I weep, but I'm glad to have them!

New dreams now excite me.
New activities fill old gaps.
I shall survive.

Bonnie Johannes
March, 1986